M000283485

"With vulnerability and much-needed insights th... ... painful experiences, all while looking to the One who 'heals the brokenhearted, and binds up their wounds' (Psalm 147:3). This book will impart hope as you walk out your journey of healing in Jesus Christ!"

Dr. Ché Ahn, president, Harvest International Ministry;
senior pastor, Harvest Rock Church, Pasadena, California;
international chancellor, Wagner University

"Dr. Mark Chironna has a one-of-a-kind mind, with unmatched focus on God's Word, His people, and the advancement of His Kingdom. Yet he is human and faces some of the same struggles and devastations we all do. The bravery to document and re-count for us his painful journey through some of his darkest days is inspiring. God knew He could trust him, like Job, to come out on the other side giving God all of the glory!"

Pastor Sheryl Brady, The Potter's House of North Dallas

"A raw and honest discussion of Mark Chironna's struggle to overcome anxiety and deep depression. Mark blends together his background in theology, psychology, and pastoral ministry in addressing these battles. He reminds us that, ultimately, it is not a technique that will deliver us, but the person of Jesus Christ."

Dr. Michael L. Brown, radio host, *Line of Fire*;
author, *Has God Failed You?*

"I saw Mark Chironna enter his 'valley of the shadow of death' and saw his self-awareness and God-awareness intersect in pain-ful ways. Without making excuses or tangential reasoning, my good friend Mark shares with you his life, his losses, his regain-ing his sight and finding God in refreshing ways. You'll love this book and share it with all you know."

Sam Chand, leadership architect, consultant, author

"Mark Chironna's *On the Edge of Hope* is a powerful book that speaks to the reality of the dark side of emotional, spiritual, and psychological breakdown. Mark's honesty regarding his struggle was powerful. The challenges his dark night of the soul brought to his charismatic Pentecostal theology and how the experience reoriented some of his theology were insightful and helpful. I highly recommend it!"

Dr. Randy Clark, founder and president,
Apostolic Network of Global Awakening

"The growing urgency for transparency in our culture is indicative of the things we've given power to by keeping them hidden. When leaders embrace this vulnerable obligation to humanity, they inspire hope in the hearts of those who might otherwise have succumbed to the dark. Dr. Mark Chironna brilliantly invites us to venture beyond the pretense of hypocrisy, where we are empowered to conquer lies and live on the edge of discovery. Get ready to believe again!"

Brenda Crouch, author, speaker, TV host

"I passed through the valley of the shadow of death that Psalm 23 speaks about at the same time a dear friend quietly suffered through an extended dark night of the soul. We identified with one another. We had few answers except to say, 'Keep your hand on the plow and look straight ahead.' My friend was none other than Mark Chironna. Thank you, Mark, for being transparent and brave and walking a path less beaten."

James W. Goll, God Encounters Ministries;
GOLL Ideation LLC

"It's hard to tell the truth about what we've suffered. It's even harder to tell the truth in ways that awaken genuine hope (and not wishful thinking). But Mark Chironna has done that. Precisely because he hasn't glossed over any of his pains, God's goodness shines through every line."

Chris E. W. Green, professor of public theology,
Southeastern University

"As spiritual leaders, we often carry the burden of our sheep upon our shoulders, even in the midst of going through our personal struggles and battles. I am so grateful to Mark Chironna for penning his darkest season of pain. His sharing about his innermost thoughts and struggles while going through the darkest season of his life will be an encouragement to many as we witness the goodness and reality of God in his life. All glory to God!"

Rev. Kong Hee, founder and senior pastor,
City Harvest Church, Singapore

"Bishop Chironna has given the Body of Christ a precious and costly gift—the testimony of his three and a half years of suffering. He masterfully weaves together personal stories, psychological analysis, and deep theological reflection. Those suffering their own dark night of the soul will find this book to be a compassionate, nonjudgmental, and hopeful companion. Chironna also serves as a guide to those who minister to people suffering from depression, grief, and anxiety. It is well-researched but written on a lay level."

Cheryl Bridges Johns, senior professor of discipleship and
Christian formation, Pentecostal Theological Seminary

"Suffering is real. Perhaps we have forgotten God's compassionate solidarity with those who suffer and are brokenhearted. Mark Chironna's *On the Edge of Hope* brings us to remembrance with a scriptural and Spirit-led theology of suffering illustrated by his own painful journey to hope and healing. Pass it on."

Rev. Kim Maas, MDiv, DMin, author,
Prophetic Community and *The Way of the Kingdom*

"Familiar with the edge of despair and paralyzing pain, Mark Chironna is also at home in the landscape of honest hope and healing love. In the company of Jesus, Job, Jung, et al., Mark humbly offers truth and wisdom gained through the suffering and renewal of his own life."

Dr. Cherith Fee Nordling, theologian

"Balanced tenuously on the cusp of despair and hope, one can turn one way and see nothing but darkness. Dr. Chironna summons us to turn and look instead at the boundless sea of hope. I strongly recommend this powerful and authentic work on inner healing."

Mark Rutland, executive director,
National Institute of Christian Leadership

"A monumental book of sweeping wisdom and weeping compassion. Mark Chironna has composed a manifesto of hope that conveys both modesty of spirit and majesty of thought. A remarkable achievement."

Leonard Sweet, professor; publisher;
founder, PreachTheStory.com;
author, Songs of Light series

"*On the Edge of Hope* offers a lifeline to those drowning in a sea of depression or anxiety. Through Mark's personal healing journey, you will find a lighthouse in the midst of your storm that will guide you to the shores of peace and help you win the battle against hopelessness. I highly recommend this book to anyone who is going through a storm or knows someone who is!"

Kris Vallotton, senior associate leader, Bethel Church,
Redding, California; cofounder, Bethel School of
Supernatural Ministry; author, *The Supernatural Ways of
Royalty*, *Heavy Rain*, *Spiritual Intelligence*, and more

ON THE

EDGE
OF
HOPE

ON THE
EDGE
OF
HOPE

NO MATTER HOW
DARK THE NIGHT, THE
REDEEMED SOUL *still* SINGS

MARK CHIRONNA

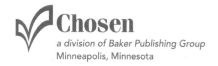
Chosen
a division of Baker Publishing Group
Minneapolis, Minnesota

Published by Chosen Books
11400 Hampshire Avenue South
Minneapolis, Minnesota 55438
www.chosenbooks.com

Chosen Books is a division of
Baker Publishing Group, Grand Rapids, Michigan

Printed in the United States of America

Library of Congress Cataloging-in-Publication Data
Names: Chironna, Mark, author.
Title: On the edge of hope : no matter how dark the night, the redeemed soul still sings / Mark Chironna.
Description: Minneapolis, Minnesota : Chosen Books, a division of Baker Publishing Group, [2022] | Includes bibliographical references.
Identifiers: LCCN 2022004694 | ISBN 9780800762575 (trade paper) | ISBN 9780800762995 (casebound) | ISBN 9781493437481 (ebook)
Subjects: LCSH: Suffering—Religious aspects—Christianity. | Pain—Religious aspects—Christianity. | Hope—Religious aspects—Christianity.
Classification: LCC BV4909 .C45 2022 | DDC 248.8/6—dc23/eng/20220225
LC record available at https://lccn.loc.gov/2022004694

To
Reverend Vincent Bernard Manzo,
without whose help, wisdom, guidance, and presence my
dark season would have been utterly intolerable

Contents

Foreword

What started out as a fun family ski trip turned into my being strapped to a stretcher in the back of an ambulance on my way to the hospital. One moment I was skiing downhill, the next I was in the air in an unplanned somersault listening to a *pop-pop-pop* come from my right knee. I had snapped my ACL, torn my MCL and meniscus, and fractured my knee. Never had I experienced that kind of pain. In the days following, I hobbled around with a leg brace and crutches until I could have surgery for a hamstring graft.

I was still in the recovery room when a physical therapist said, "Chris, you did a lot of damage to your knee, and most people tend to not fully recover after that sort of injury. It's not that you can't recover, because, thanks to surgery, your right knee is now technically stronger than your left knee, but the challenge is whether you will be willing to endure the recovery process. The injury happened suddenly and quickly, but the recovery process will take several months of focused and painful therapy. There is no way to avoid the pain. You can recover fully or partially, quickly or slowly—it will be totally up to you. The degree to which you are willing to embrace the recovery process is the degree to which you will recover and thrive again."

These were not words I wanted to hear after a painful, traumatic accident, nor was the process one I necessarily wanted to endure. But if I wanted to get well, if I wanted to be able to run again, do squats, even ski, then I had to agree to go through the process of recovery. I would have done anything for a friend with the gift of healing to come and lay hands on me and for me to instantaneously jump out of bed, fully healed, and run laps of praise around the hospital. Alas, although many people did pray for me, there was no instantaneous miracle. If I wanted to be able to move my knee again, I was going to have to go through the process of healing. Little did I realize how much I would have to suffer to be able to experience healing.

I don't have the words to express the pain involved in breaking up the scar tissue at a cellular level in my knee and learning to walk, run, and yes, even ski again. The physical therapy required to prevent a collection of tough, fibrous tissue from interfering with my mobility involved repeated stretching, strategic exercises, and other treatments, to the point I thought I couldn't bear it. Every move was excruciating, the recovery long, but the results in ensuring a great quality of life in my second half was more than worth it.

Could God have intervened and miraculously and instantaneously healed my leg? And delivered me from all my pain? Of course, and I've seen God do such miracles in other people's lives, but in my case, He allowed me to go through a recovery process that involved pain, suffering, and endurance. Looking back, I have rarely felt closer to Him or more dependent upon Him than when I have been in such trying times.

What's more, it has not only been in the physical realm that I have gone through a process of recovery to find healing and wholeness, but also in the realm of my wounded soul, broken heart, and tormented mind. I come from a background of abandonment, adoption, and sexual abuse. I have carried a lot of spiritual and psychological "scar tissue" around in years past because of things that happened to me when I was not even old enough to understand what was happening to me. I have come to understand that because we live in a fallen world, bad things can and do happen to good people. No one can escape the effects of a fallen world. Jesus Himself said that in this world we *will* have troubles (see John 16:33). He did not say if we have enough faith then we won't have any trouble; He gave no exemption. Therefore, we should not be surprised that troubles, pain, suffering, and varying degrees of trauma and injustice are part of this life.

The real problem is not that these things are a part of life, but that we do not know how to walk in faith and simultaneously wrestle with profound pain. We often have a faulty belief system that tells us we need to deny, dismiss, or diminish our pain or suffering in order to live victorious, overcoming Christian lives. We often feel like failures because we have tried to declare, decree, and confess victory and freedom with no tangible change in our life or circumstances. We have tried all the formulas, prayed all the prayers, attended all the conferences, sowed all our seed, tried to fake it by faith until we make it, and nothing has seemed to work. Despite our best efforts, we still feel bound, broken, tormented, anxious, distressed, or depressed. We wonder, *Where is this abundant life Jesus promised? Where is the victory? Where is the freedom? Where is the joy? Where is the peace? Where is the hope?*

I believe the book you are holding in your hands answers such wondering. I believe it will be one of the most important books you are ever going to read. Dr. Chironna masterfully integrates the theological with the psychological as he teaches us how to wrestle with the complexities of the human condition. As he takes us into the journey of Job, we discover that we can accept the mystery of suffering and not be ashamed of our own suffering. And that absolutely any one of us can stand strong in one moment and struggle the next; it is simply part of living in a fallen world. The good news is we can all learn to trust ourselves to the goodness of God, who loves us perfectly, even when the process of sanctification does not always feel good in the moment.

My physical therapist wanted my knee to have full range of motion and for me to be able to do any and all activities, so I had to go through the painful recovery process. Everything in me wanted to avoid the rehabilitation, skip sessions, and be instantly healed, but I had to stick with it, day after day, week after week, and month after month, to be where I am today. I encourage you not to try to run from your pain, ruminate on your past, or fear your future. Do the work, answer the questions at the end of each chapter, sit at the feet of Jesus, and yield to the process of sanctification. It is there you will find healing, wholeness, and freedom. It is there you will be spiritually formed and transformed. It is there you will discover you are truly known, seen, and fully loved. It is there you will experience your belovedness that is only found in Him.

Christine Caine

Acknowledgments

When it comes to writing a book, the task, at least for me, has never been a small undertaking. I am ever grateful for the support of my wife, Ruth, and her encouragement, her prayers, and her willingness to sacrifice her time with me for time with writing. She is a trooper, and after all these years is used to the process. She has exhibited great grace in giving me space to take on this challenge and opportunity, for which I am forever grateful. The dark season I experienced was something she had to endure with me, all while we learned to face life's day-to-day affairs with faith, courage, stamina, and fortitude, for the sake of our children and the church we pioneered.

I want to thank my son Matthew for the way he has supported me as he travels with me on the road and has gotten used to a dad who is always either writing on the plane or writing in the hotel, and then having to speak at various conferences. My writing takes place mostly while he is quietly being a caring presence with me during all my ministry time away from home. He never complains, he is always available for whatever I need, and he always anticipates what I may need without me having to ask.

Thank you to my daughter-in-law, Ashley, for allowing her husband to travel with me and give up time with her and the children, because she knows that in all of this God is at work in mostly hidden but sometimes obvious ways.

Thanks goes to my son Daniel for all he has taught me about overcoming insurmountable odds, his will to survive from his earliest struggles, and how in spite of all those struggles, he has continued to persevere.

Many thanks also to my four grandchildren for the constant joy and inspiration they are to me. Ariana, Mark, Londyn, and Enzo—each one holds a very special and treasured place in my heart. It is hard to explain how they have given me great joy, during and since my dark season, in a way that words cannot describe.

I also want to thank Misty Hood, my administrative pastor, for her tireless willingness not only to administrate the process of this project along with everything else on her plate, but also to take up all the slack with managing my schedule, my appointments, and all the nitty-gritty details of making sure the staff at Chosen Books has consistent and timely communication and approvals. Writing this book during the final stages of postgraduate work on another doctoral degree has required her to make sure I stick to a rigid schedule. She has managed that and me well. During that dark season, when the best I could do was manage to preach on Sundays and at our midweek services, she had the responsibility of keeping the church running on an even keel. She did a masterful job.

I want to thank my entire pastoral staff at Church on the Living Edge for the way they have trusted me not only when things have gone well, but also when I felt quite incapable. They all rose to the occasion and made the rough places smooth.

I want to thank Donna Scuderi, as she has been such a help in making sure my voice stays intact when my words get ahead of my thoughts and need be corralled. Donna had to do double duty during the writing of this book, as she has edited all my thesis work, as well as the first half of the book you now hold in your hands. I am grateful for who she is to me personally, to our entire church family, and to the Body of Christ at large.

I also want to thank Dr. Chris E. W. Green, who, in a moment when Donna's tasks grew far more monumental than we both realized, willingly stepped in and finished editing my manuscript, paying careful attention to the details and being faithful to my intent in every sentence and paragraph he scoured.

I also want to thank Kim Bangs at Chosen Books for her ceaseless encouragement and prayers as I was moving through this process to bring the book to completion. She has made this journey an absolute joy, and she has been a solid prayer partner who covered me as I found spots in the writing that triggered pain to revisit.

I am deeply grateful for Ginger Kolbaba, Chosen's editor for this book, for the way she worked through the manuscript with an eye for grasping what I intended to say, helping me perfect the way I said it, and assuring that readers would be able to grasp it and make it applicable in their lives. She is a gem.

I want to thank the entire Church on the Living Edge family, who, through their ongoing inspiration to me in good times and bad, have made pastoring a joy that I wouldn't trade for the world, and who in that darkest season of my life never gave up on me. They are my heart.

Finally, I am deeply humbled that Christine Caine would consent to write the foreword for this book. I am always amazed at how Providence works in our lives, how God serendipitously places people in our pathway who make such a profound difference in more ways than words can tell. God has graced Christine with a measure of wisdom and faith that is an inspiration to all of us. It is an honor to call her "friend."

Introduction

If I'd Seen the Bus Coming . . .

> For everything there is an appointed time . . . a time to bear and
> a time to die . . . a time to weep and a time to laugh; a time to
> mourn and a time to dance; a time to throw away stones and
> a time to gather stones . . . a time to seek and a time to lose.
>
> Ecclesiastes 3:1–2, 4–6 LEB

Reflecting on a certain prolonged dark season of my life, I often
say, "If I had seen the bus coming, I would have gotten out of
the way!" The truth is that even if I had seen it coming, it would
have been too late. That bus was headed my way for some time.
When it finally hit me, it did so with full force and no qualms
about the effects on my well-being or that of my loved ones.

The ensuing dark season brought deep psychological and
physical suffering. For three and a half years, the anxiety persisted, and depression came along for the ride. I had no rest
and virtually no sleep, day or night. It is difficult to describe
the damage from that kind of sleep deprivation. You know you
are in for a rough ride when your anxiety keeps your eyes from

closing. Medical experts say that the body will eventually fall asleep, but that did not happen in my case.

I don't share these details from a place of self-pity. My concern is the reality of human suffering and its implications for Christians and non-Christians alike. When the bus hit me, I was a Christian. In fact, I was on a ministry trip far from home, where I planned to preach to thousands of people who wanted answers for their own struggles. How ironic! I thought providing answers for others was my role, but I arrived at the venue weighed down by some very hard questions of my own.

I reached a well-traveled crossroad that day—the same one many people reach every day. Mine brought me face-to-face with unconscious drivers operating deep within my heart and mind. Although the crisis came as a shock, the conditions preceding it were common. A certain amount of unfinished business drives the emotions, feelings, and behaviors of all human beings. It is often the residue of our earliest years of formation and life. As grown-ups, we are not fully conscious of all that adolescence instilled in us. Much of it remains unresolved. Often, it returns to haunt us in our *middlessence*, the period from our thirties through our sixties.

You might be at a similar crossroad right now. It may be difficult to explain your pain to others and even harder to process it for yourself. That is why I wrote this book. None of us—not preachers, doctors, movie stars, philosophers, or even self-help gurus—are exempt from the kind of suffering that seems to come out of nowhere. Even the people who appear to have it "all together" can experience indescribable challenges. Whether we expect them or believe they cannot touch us, those challenges are part of the human condition. They may be preventable, not because we deny their existence or believe we are spiritually inoculated against them, but because we become attuned to our unfinished business and deal with it before it deals with us.

I do not offer the questions and insights in these pages as therapy but as confirmation that we humans have an awful lot in common and can benefit from being transparent about our struggles. Although I have a long history of training in psychology and theology, this book comes out of a long period of processing what my dark place revealed. I have learned some things about

> » what led me into the path of the cosmic "bus" I mentioned earlier;
> » how my beliefs contributed to or exacerbated my suffering;
> » how those beliefs tailored my responses to suffering, and how those responses helped or hindered my healing; and
> » what the Bible really says about suffering and about our psychology.

These are some of the things I feel called to share. They don't come from any sense of having arrived or excelled above anyone else. They aren't theoretical or designed to tickle your ears. They come from a place of realizing how precious life is and how much we need God's help to live each day. I know I could not have survived my dark season without Him, and I am forever grateful that He kept me, even when I believed my suffering would never end.

Time to Get Real

In case you haven't noticed, lots of folks you know are either hiding their pain or doing their best to process it. We are all in the same boat: Nobody was raised in a perfect environment by perfect people, and nobody is perfect. We are all somewhat dysfunctional, precisely because of what Christians acknowledge as the Adamic Fall. Sin makes us vulnerable to brokenness, and our brokenness increases our vulnerability to suffering. Yet, in Christ, we are acceptable before God. He has imputed His righteousness to us. But we are still sinners (see Romans 7:14–20). Therefore, Christ is in the business, by the Spirit, of putting our lives back together again. He is continually remembering us and returning us to the Father's original intent, which is to make us more human.

We cannot separate our journey to humanness from the need to face our brokenness, fragility, vulnerabilities, pains, and sins. From beginning to end, God's perfect love works to reveal our humanness in its fullness. His work will continue until we receive our resurrected bodies. Until then, we hope against hope, even amid our suffering and pain, knowing that God is not the author of evil and cannot commit it. God did not ordain the bus that ran over me. But, sure enough, it ran me down.

Maybe you can relate to my experience. Really, I believe anyone who has lived more than a few years can relate in some measure. We have all heard stories of people who were standing strong one moment and struggling the next. Things happen that we do not fully understand, but we need not be ashamed of them. And we certainly should not ignore them. What we can do is accept the mystery of suffering and realize that all of us will taste of it at some point in our lives.

I once knew a precious woman, a highly skilled nurse who served as a nutritionist. She dedicated her professional life to colon health and worked with doctors on behalf of her clients and patients. She provided my wife and me tremendous help when we faced digestive concerns. Gracious and kind and always the picture of health, she had a flawless complexion and clear, bright eyes. Her beautiful smile filled the room.

One afternoon I had a luncheon appointment in the city where we lived at the time. As I finished lunch and walked toward the exit of the restaurant, I saw this woman sitting alone in one of the booths. Her countenance was fallen. Her amazing complexion had a gray pallor. When I stopped to say hello and ask about her well-being, she began to weep.

The woman who meticulously guarded the colon health and well-being of so many people had contracted colon cancer herself. Late in the fourth stage of the disease, doctors told her they could do nothing for her. Of course, I prayed with her and for her. She was extremely grateful. The irony of her situation struck me: A woman whose career centered on colon health suffered the ravages of colon disease! It left me shaking my head.

In a matter of weeks, this dear woman passed into eternity. Her life had not unfolded in a predictable way. Very few lives do. Doctors get sick, psychologists sometimes need to see other psychologists, and pastors and leaders who care for the souls of others suffer from afflictions in their own souls.

Life's paradoxes are all around us, and human suffering is ubiquitous, whether we want to admit it or not. All of us battle at times with distressing or overwhelming negative thoughts, emotions, and feelings. On the surface, some people seem to handle them better than others. But do they? What about you? How have you handled your seasons of stress and pain? Will you be honest enough to say, "I probably could have handled it better"? Or would you feel too ashamed to admit it?

Either way, I understand! I grappled with these issues and know that some of my responses to pain hurt me more than they helped me. I understand why people work so hard to conceal their suffering. They don't want other people to think something is wrong with them. But, beloved, there is "something wrong" with all of us. We live in a fallen, sin-stained world, and we all suffer its effects—yes, even those of us who call Jesus Christ our Lord and Savior. Why else would we *need* a Savior?

Speaking from the perspective of the Church, are we not called to come alongside those who suffer? Or are we called to selectively judge the suffering of others and even reject those whose sufferings seem in some way taboo to us? Is *that* our theology?

I am eternally grateful to those who stood by me in my dark season and spoke life into my breaking heart. I did not need anyone to judge me or give me the "answers." I spent plenty of time judging myself and trying to figure out why I was going through hell. Instead, I needed reminders that I was God's beloved. I needed someone to tell me that we all suffer, and our suffering does not last forever. Whether they realized it or not, the people who did these things helped me climb out of the depths and live. They did not succumb to covering up, ignoring, or shaming. They recognized that my struggle was real, and they were real with me. It made all the difference!

The Wake-Up Call

If I learned anything from my dark season, I learned to pay attention! Prior to July 2007, I was "blowing and going," as the expression goes. My rigorous schedule included flying four or five times a week, speaking in four or five places, plus heading the local church where I was pastor. I also did one-on-one certified coaching and group coaching. I earned a psychology degree and continued to study theology. Each month, I read a minimum of fifteen books, and I managed to get by on four or five hours of sleep each night. Meanwhile, I dealt with the usual issues that face the parents of teenagers, and I was navigating our church's move into a larger, more expensive building.

I had a lot on my plate! From the outside looking in, you might have thought I was "successful." In some ways, I thought so too. For years, I had managed to keep up that kind of schedule without blinking an eye. But I wasn't paying attention to the fatigue in my body or how tense I was becoming. I had a bout with heart palpitations that sent me to a cardiologist.

A series of tests over the course of several weeks proved that nothing was wrong with my heart. But I *was* carrying a lot on my shoulders—and not handling it as well as I thought.

By the time July 2007 arrived, the cosmic bus had caught up with me. It was the wake-up call I could not ignore. I have more to tell you about that season, but for now, I will say that by the grace of God, I lived to tell the story. To borrow the words of Maya Angelou, I "wouldn't take nothing for my journey now." As difficult as my hard time was, I would not trade it or what I learned from it.

My Hope and Prayer

While I can lay claim to a master's degree in psychology, I am not a clinical specialist. Likewise, despite my doctorate in theology, I do not have God all figured out. In fact, I contend that the more I learn about the human psyche and the Triune God, I concur with the apostle Paul, who said, "We know only in part" (1 Corinthians 13:9). Whatever I say in these pages or anywhere else can only be "in part." I do not have all the answers.

My prayer as you read this book, however, is that God will use it as a vehicle to empower you. I have shared everything I could share, and I pray that it will help you as you learn to navigate your pain and suffering, particularly the kind of pain and suffering you experience as negative, distressing, and over-whelming thoughts, emotions, feelings, and moods. I also want to encourage you to realize that you might need more support than this book can provide. There is no shame in needing the services of a well-trained helping professional. As a Christian leader, I thought there was—until I needed help myself. I realize now that my prior approach was less than authentic. In God's mercy, my suffering drew me out of my misunderstanding of the Jesus who loves and cares for us deeply. In time, I realized that the One who gave His life for us is not the least bit ashamed when we get the help we need.

What is more important than any baseless taboo is that you come to know—truly *know*—deep in your interior that Jesus loves you so fully and completely that He will be with you in the darkest, most seemingly God-forsaken emotional places. The history of His love attests to this truth! When Jesus crossed the Kidron Valley and entered the Garden of Gethsemane to pray to His Father, He allowed Himself to experience the deep suffering and agony of our forsakenness. It was there that He Himself despaired of life. In His humanness, He wrestled with the very things that confound us (see Mark 14:32–36; Luke 22:39–44).

Jesus knows what your suffering and my suffering are like. With that in mind, I invite you to take a healing journey through these pages. What I will share is like me—far from perfect. My focus, however, is the truths that brought me through a very long and distressing season. Jesus is the One who perfects us, day by day. The same Jesus lifted me out from under the bus and stood me back on my feet. Because of Him, I can say, "Surely goodness and mercy shall follow me all the days of my life" (Psalm 23:6 NKJV)!

1

How Did I Get Here?

> Living with anxiety is like being followed by a voice. It knows
> all your insecurities and uses them against you. It gets to the
> point when it's the loudest voice in the room. The only one
> you can hear.
>
> Anonymous

When the bus is coming at you, getting out of the way seems like a solution. But can you avoid getting hit by something you refuse to see? My experience with crushing anxiety tells me that you cannot. Looking back, I chose to compartmentalize the signs that presented themselves. I convinced myself that I would deal with them "when I had the time." Whatever was brewing, it would have to keep until my schedule eased up.

When the pressure is on, procrastination can seem like a great way to bury your problems. The underlying, unspoken hope is that they will eventually take care of themselves. The truth is that whatever you bury alive stays alive and burrows deeper into your heart. Postponing your attention feels comforting, but only for the moment. The issues you avoid will only fester until you face them.

Trust me when I say we can convince ourselves that we are dealing with reality when we are not. The prophet Jeremiah wrote that "the heart is more deceitful than all else" and intimated that we don't even understand it (Jeremiah 17:9 NASB). In other words, our hearts can play tricks on us. I learned this truth the hard way. When I ignored the signs of trouble ahead, I conveniently split what was real from what I wanted to think was real. I created a bubble of magical thinking in which I could isolate myself from the problem and conjure a false sense of security, a façade that said, *Everything is fine.*

That kind of thinking feels good, but not for long. There was no escaping the underlying issues. The longer I ignored them, the more powerful they became. They were bound to surface, regardless of my schedule and commitments. The fact that I was busy and keeping up with my schedule did not prove that I was fine. My issues kept brewing despite my formidable schedule.

When the bus finally hit me, panic ensued. It came as I followed my busy schedule and traveled to a pulpit far from home. Despite my sudden agony, I would have to preach as though everything was okay.

Facing the Unthinkable

When panic comes, it comes in disorienting, debilitating waves. The first wave hit me at thirty-two thousand feet above the Atlantic. All hell seemed to break loose, as though the ocean below had released a torrent to tear me apart, inside and out. In terms of pain, I had little to compare it with other than a bout of kidney stones years earlier. Those stones also hit with full force! I remember thinking that passing out would be a godsend. At least I would get a break from the pain. But I never did pass out, and the pain never subsided. To get at the source, I had to take medication and have an operation.

Anxiety is different. You cannot cut out the source of your emotional anguish. Instead, you must face it. But facing it was the last thing I wanted. Amid the suffering, I prayed for a normal night's sleep—or any sleep at all. And when the anxiety was the most intense (which it was for most of the next 1,278 days), the idea of falling asleep and never waking up sounded like mercy to me. Thankfully, I did not enter my final sleep. But neither did I find the nightly escape of slumber. The anxiety would not release me into any significant period of shut-eye.

What I faced in the Caribbean at the very beginning of my dark season was like nothing I had ever known. I thought I was having a panic attack and assumed it would end in a reasonable amount of time. Instead, it became a fixed and unrelenting anxiety that soon teamed up with depression. The condition was tough enough, but it produced a psychological and physiological feedback loop that was 100 percent negative, which only made things worse. For the entirety of the ordeal, I had almost no break from the fight-or-flight response. In fact, I experienced no rest of any kind at all.

Enter the accuser of the brethren, the expert exploiter. He used the beautiful promise that says "he gives sleep to his beloved" as a torment and accusation to me (Psalm 127:2)—a torment because I could not grasp why a loving God had overlooked my prayer for relief, and an accusation because the powers of darkness twisted God's promise and convinced me that I was under judgment in some area of my life. Whether I was my worst enemy or the devil was, I did not know. But I felt as though I had been engulfed and swallowed up by evil.

I felt that it had conquered me and God had forsaken me. The darkness was very dark. The trauma was all too real, too endless, and utterly unthinkable.

Magical Thinking

During my dark season, nothing would have been more welcome than an instantaneous healing or a Scripture verse to "zap" whatever demon had descended upon me. When months and years passed without either form of deliverance, I learned the hardest lesson of my life—one I'm still learning. It shattered my misconceptions about Scripture and about God Himself. Everything I thought I believed was tested, and many misguided views were stripped away. Much of what I believed involved the magical thinking I mentioned earlier. Like many other followers of Jesus in a consumer-driven culture, I bought into some unproven, unsound ideas that could not help me when the bus showed up.

Beloved, I heard all the barn-burning messages and even preached some of them! I read all the books and "knew" all the techniques about how to be free, get healed, and defeat demons. I understood what it was to lay hands on the sick and see them recover. I still do! Healing *is* the children's bread, but that does not mean we will never suffer or face trials.

Many popular Christian teachings lead us to think in magical ways that have little to do with scriptural truth. Therefore, they have almost nothing to do with spiritual formation and transformation. We accept them because we like the idea of three easy steps and a quick way out of our struggles.

As the popular psychologist Dr. Phil would say, "How's that working for you?" My point is that if it had worked, none of us would be facing the issues before us. None of us would ever be sick or financially strapped. None of us would die of cancer or heart disease. And none of us would suffer bouts of emotional and psychological turmoil. If our magical thinking were effective, none of us would be searching for yet another quick fix.

Perhaps the worst part of our reliance on magical formulas is that we sacrifice the genuine article, which is to know the truth experientially and deeply and to allow it to bring us into real freedom. *That* is the wholeness we really need and want. The problem we have with the genuine article is that it rarely brings instant relief—what we most yearn for when our suffering seems unbearable.

Avoidance Strategies

Before my season of trouble came, I ignored its warning signs. The mind can do a pretty good job of burying the evidence, but we pay a price on the back end. The price of my avoidance was a perpetual fight-or-flight posture that I thought might never end. Having deftly ignored my body's warning system, I now faced its ultimate response: more than forty months on full alert, without sleep, rest, appetite, or peace, and barely able to lower my eyelids. It was a brutal combination of anxiety and depression. Yet even after the onset of my anxiety, my avoidance strategies continued.

Some of them were more subtle than others. I developed one strategy from a very logical question: "How did I ever get here?" I rightly wanted to know how and why the bus came after me. Maybe if I figured out where it came from, I could send it back and forget it ever happened. Or maybe I could control the thing. I'm not entirely sure what I was thinking. Of course, the issue was not as simple as I tried to make it. In fact, it proved to be much more complicated.

Each of us has a different temperament. We are unique personalities, and we process our pain differently. I tend to be analytical and pensive. When I think about something, I consider it from every conceivable angle. That is what I did with my question about "how I got here." The question seemed logical enough. If I wanted to understand where I was, I needed to figure out where I had been.

For someone as deeply analytical and pensive as I am, however, a simple overview was not going to be enough (at least not in my mind). So my analysis quickly turned into endless rumination. I chewed over my past almost ceaselessly. I know now that ruminating about anxiety and depression is not helpful to our well-being or hope for the future because it leads to "awful-izing." The more we think about how terrible we feel, the worse we feel. And when we reflect on our past from our current place of pain, our minds automatically select the memories that confirm the "awfulness." Instead of figuring out how we got into our current crisis, we end up reconstructing in the present moment the pains we remember from our past—and even projecting them into our future.

The fact is that all memory is reconstructed. Nobody remembers events exactly as they happened. Instead, we remember them as they seemed to us, based on our way of seeing and understanding the world. We don't like the idea that we reconstruct our memories, but we have no other way to recall a past that no longer exists. To remember it is to re-member or reconstruct it.

Accepting this reality and realizing that our memories are not entirely trustworthy are essential components of mental health. The truth of reconstructed memory does not mean that we are willfully lying or making things up without any basis. Long after painful events leave indelible impressions on our psyches, we simply try to make sense of them. Because our memories are always incomplete, we naturally try to make sense of the gaps. So we fill them in with ideas that seem to emerge from the memories themselves. This "filler" comes from how we look back on events and how we process what we remember. Therefore, it is unique to us and reflects our individual ways of being.

The incompleteness of our memories probably exists for a good reason. Some scientists explain it from the perspective of evolutionary biology. From a theological perspective, we attribute it to the Fall in the Garden of Eden. The event that compromised our humanness affected every aspect of our existence and function, including our ability to cognize, perceive, imagine, remember, intuit, and reflect.

The fact is that analyzing my past and attempting to make sense of it led to an unhealthy habit of rumination. At some level, it became an avoidance strategy. If I remained fixated on remembering my past, I could avoid dealing with my current reality. In a sense, my mind tried to "pass out" and not feel the pain.

Ruminating did me much more harm than good. It is the nature of rumination that each "rehearsal" triggers new fears about our pain becoming permanent. This is partly because we battle with incomplete knowledge and faulty analysis.

Your memory is not perfect or objective. Like all of us, you assume your thoughts are 100 percent accurate because *you* are thinking them. If you are thinking about your anxiety or your insecurities, for example, you believe that every terrible thought you have is true. Then you project that negativity onto the future and ruminate on how awful tomorrow will be.

Notice that whether you are dwelling on the past or the future, you are in avoidance mode. The past is over, and you cannot retrieve or change it. And you cannot access your future because it isn't here yet. The only real space you can live in is the present moment. You cannot do it, however, with your awareness trapped in the past or the future. One of the keys that unlocks the door to freedom is to become aware of the present moment and not run from it. Yes, you can experience freedom by accepting the current moment as it is. That does not mean you surrender yourself to sickness or sorrow, for example. It means simply that you acknowledge your present state and scuttle your avoidance schemes.

Avoidance has so many painful and self-sabotaging effects. While I focused on my past and feared my future, I seemed to lack awareness of Christ's abiding presence. I knew He was always with me, yet I waited for Him to "show up" and rescue me. The blanket of anxiety and depression felt so heavy that my consciousness of Christ became marginalized. Added to that was the opportunism of the powers of darkness, with their unrelenting accusations. Some of their slanders were direct and some veiled, but they came at me day and night. (A topic worthy of another book!)

The Exempt-from-Suffering Approach

In our pain, our search for answers demands some ruthless honesty about ourselves, our beliefs, and our approach to God. When our pain seems unbearable, the last place we want to be is in the present moment. In my case, the anxiety and the stress response it triggered made me want to jump out of my skin. That seemed like the only possible way to alleviate my suffering. Of course, I knew I could not jump out and then jump back in when the storm was over.

David, the sweet psalmist of Israel, put it this way: "If I ascend to heaven, you are there! If I make my bed in Sheol, you are there!" (Psalm 139:8 ESV). All of us want to transcend our limitations and ascend into heaven. We could say it is a "sanctified way" of jumping out of our skin. David often voiced his yearning for transcendence in the immediate presence of the living God. His desire makes sense to us. Yet within his worship is this revealing proposition: "If I make my bed in Sheol . . ."

I have asked myself, "Who in their right mind would want to make their bed in hell?"

Of course, no one would *want* to. Yet all of us have made unhealthy and unwise decisions that have led to hellish consequences. The dichotomy between good and evil—even for those of us who love Jesus—runs straight through our respective beings. Some of us would disagree with such an idea. But consider the words of the apostle Paul: "I do not do the good I

How Did I Get Here?

want, but the evil I do not want is what I keep on doing" (Romans 7:19 ESV).

You might argue that Paul was speaking of his pre-conversion experience. Yet you and I and every other Christian have made sinful and foolish choices after being converted. We do not have time here for a theological exposition of pre- and post-conversion positions as they relate to Paul. The point is that he addressed what we would call a *dilatory will*—the human will that is less than perfect before God. It is the result of eating from the Tree of Knowledge of Good and Evil, which is the root of all human suffering.

If we are ruthlessly honest with ourselves, we can admit to being less than perfect before God. Our recourse is to ask His forgiveness, which explains Paul's response to his own self-sabotage. He didn't seek a technique to deliver him. He didn't cry out, "*What* shall deliver me from my mess?" Rather, he cried, "*Who* will deliver me?" (Romans 7:24 ESV). Paul did not seek a technique; he sought the Person of Christ, who loves us completely and perfectly.

To be forgiven of your sin requires you to acknowledge your sin before God. To be delivered from your pain—not through magical thinking, avoidance, running away, or any other lesser remedy—is to acknowledge your pain and take it to God. The hard part is to acknowledge and "be with" your pain. I can testify! The last thing I wanted to do when intense anxiety gripped me was to pay attention and face it. My instinct was not to accept my living hell but to run from it as fast as I could. In my agony, I could see no practical reason to do otherwise. After all, if Jesus died to set me free, I shouldn't have to go through hell in the first place! Isn't that what we think in our *Have it your way* culture? The thought of enduring and being enlarged by adversity seems nonsensical.

This became part of my strategy of pain avoidance. And when my strategies failed to work, I did not want to admit

37

their failure. I knew that ignoring the warning signs had only backfired. I knew that my avoidance did not ease my pain but only made it worse. But what else was there? Avoidance was my default response. I possessed no other well-honed response in my toolbox, except for one: the idea that if I confessed God's Word and "decreed a thing," God would wave a wand and make my pain go away—*poof!* After all, I was His child, and I wasn't *supposed* to suffer.

Today, I marvel at God's mercy toward me. He overlooked my rigidity and arrogance and brought me to the place of healing anyway. But He taught me a few things first.

The Cares of This Life

One of the great lessons of this journey involves understanding how I arrived at this difficult place. It is complicated. Life's pressures have a way of converging, even piling on at times. My bus hit me at one of those times. I cannot share all the details and all the stories, but I can say that our congregation made a move from one side of town to another. And when we did, we lost the lion's share of our membership. We also acquired a building that was far more costly than the one we sold. All of that weighed heavily on me, as it would anyone in a similar position. What made matters worse is that I believed it was all my fault. I saw it as a failure.

I didn't make any of these decisions without the counsel and support of the church leadership, of course. Still, I lived by Harry Truman's "The Buck Stops Here" rule, so I held myself totally responsible for what took place. If I were a better leader, I told myself, I would've anticipated all the worst-case scenarios and planned for them. The truth is, however, there were all kinds of unforeseeable and uncontrollable dynamics at play in those events. All at once, we were faced with the loss of our space, the need to find a suitable new building, and the stress of securing funds to buy it, as well as unethical real estate dealings, which led to lengthy legal battles.

When we finally obtained our new facility, it was on the opposite end of town. I was sure the members were so committed to the vision that they would gladly embrace the shift to another location, but many of them did not. Our first Sunday in the new building, only four hundred adults showed up—a remnant of what had been a megachurch. Additionally, the expenses of the brand-new facility far exceeded the expenses of our previous building. I found myself suddenly dealing with being the senior pastor of a much smaller congregation in a much more costly space. We had gone from a $7,000 per month mortgage to a first mortgage of $70,000 and a secondary balloon mortgage of $50,000. To put this in perspective, the mortgage on the building we sold was less than the air-conditioning bill in the new building. All of that left us with an inordinate amount of debt, and seemingly an insufficient number of congregants to manage it.

That was the beginning of unprecedented levels of anxiety in my life. And over the next several months, as we worked to create a strategy to manage the heavy mortgage, I found that what had worked in times past wasn't working now. As a result, my personal sense of incapability and incompetence increased dramatically and became overwhelming. Why hadn't God made me aware of any of this in time for me to have made better decisions? Had I failed to regard the voice of the Lord?

I will talk more about perplexity later, but at this juncture in my life perplexity was all around me. As it laid a more total claim over my mind, my emotions, my feelings, and even my body, I became more and more apprehensive. How were we going to make ends meet? Because I feared the house would buckle and fold, my mind had a difficult time focusing on study or prayer. Thus, the preparation and delivery of timely, substantive messages that would feed the flock proved increasingly hard. Having lost so many people in the move, I was bound by fear that the financial burden would sooner or later cause the remnant to leave as well, so that in the end we would lose everything we had ever worked for.

Although I was incredibly apprehensive, I managed for a while to hold up under the stress because I worked out regularly and hard. After the bus hit, however, the anxiety was simply too much. I was totally in the dark, constantly bewildered. My thoughts started to have me instead of me having them. As Russ Harris, a trainer in the acceptance and commitment therapy model, says, I was being "pushed around,"[1] bullied by negative thoughts and feelings and emotions.

This complex scenario played a part in my experience with anxiety and depression. In His goodness, however, God helped me to understand the dynamics of the experience so that I could learn and grow in the process.

But let me say this before I say anything else: We all learn at our own pace. The pain for me was so great that it took me a while to learn. I say this not to discourage you, but in hopes that it will help you recognize where you are and what is happening to you. I trust my story can help you learn more quickly than I did, so the disentangling can happen as it should. Let me be clear: I was the reason for the delay, not God. And God was never impatient with me, even when I was impatient with myself. God was faithful, as God always is. And He saw me through the darkness.

Out of the Bubble

In the words of John Newton, "I once . . . was blind, but now I see!"[2] Really, my "sight" is still being adjusted. But I can honestly say that my long, dark season changed me. Not only do I understand how I arrived at such a crossroad, but the experience tested my beliefs and weeded out some fallacious ones. Today, I read the Scriptures differently. I wrestle with them more. I ask more questions about things I seem to know and things I don't. I'm more open to certain ideas than I was before I was tested. I hear people and their pain far more acutely. I discern their trauma more precisely. I sense their suffering in a deeper way. My pressing through and beyond my own pain has brought me closer to the One who ever stands as the Paschal Lamb, having been freshly slain on the throne of the universe (see Revelation 5:6). For all of this, I am eternally grateful!

Two centuries ago, Christ followers thought it wise to be wary of psychological theory. Much needful work has been done in the past century and a half, however. Brilliant thinkers who love Jesus and desire to integrate the psychological with the theological have impacted the world of therapeutic consciousness. I believe that integrating the best of these disciplines will bring healing and hope to people in pain—those who didn't see the bus coming and are now pressing through the long, dark aftermath.

Let's face facts: Our thinking is not always as sound as we would like it to be. Far too many issues, events, and experiences of human suffering impact us. We live in a culture where everyone wants to win all the time. So the people who lose feel like they don't belong. We tend to think that Jesus hangs out with winners. I would argue that far more often, He hangs out with folks who have suffered loss or been disenfranchised, disillusioned, distressed, and downcast, like sheep without a shepherd.

Beloved, there is a Wonderful Counselor who knows the soul's dark night firsthand. Strangely enough, through my valley of shadows, I got to know Him in a way I never had before. Trust me: There were many shadows, and they haunted me at every turn—morning, noon, and night.

You may be in that valley right now. Maybe you used to be or feel that you might be headed there. Whatever your situation, I can promise you that, with God, the end of the matter is better than the beginning (see Ecclesiastes 7:8). I can also promise that even when your trial feels like a life sentence, it is only a season. I cannot tell you how long that the season will last, but I know that when you cry out, "How long, LORD? Will You forget me forever?" (Psalm 13:1 NASB), God is there.

I often think about the words of the great Dr. Charles S. Price, the Pentecostal pioneer and healing evangelist. I have heard hundreds of his sermons and remember him saying that the redeemed soul continues to sing, even in the dark night.[3] In my dark night, I had to learn how to sing. I was already trained vocally and had an undergraduate degree in music and performance. But when pain consumed me, I had to take singing lessons from the Holy Spirit. They were lessons in the naked faith that held when nothing seemed to work, and God seemed to turn a blind eye to my suffering.

Whatever your story may be, you can learn to sing! However feebly you might start out, you can endure your dark season and know that it *will* end. You will come out the other side with something only God could give you, and no one can take away.

QUESTIONS TO PONDER

» What fears can you identify in your life that keep cropping up?

» Where do you find you hesitate most when it comes to making decisions?

» Can you identify those areas in your life where you tend to avoid facing situations or things that trigger painful thoughts and emotions? What are they?

2

Acceptance Is Not
a Dirty Word

Be content with who you are, and don't put on airs. God's
strong hand is on you.

1 Peter 5:6 MSG

At this moment, you and I are somewhere in our respective
journeys. It is not where we have always been or where we
will always be. We are headed somewhere we have not yet been.
Even if we have a sense of what that place is, we cannot know
it fully until the time comes. But what we can know is where we
are right now. Accepting that is a major key to our well-being.

Through many years of ministry, I have traveled through almost every one of these United States. In the early days, flying to
multiple speaking engagements wasn't affordable, so my wife,
Ruth, and I drove from place to place, clocking countless miles
and crisscrossing the nation again and again. The interstates

43

showed us how vast the country is and how long it can take to travel from point A to point B. I can remember starting a trip in Bergen County, New Jersey, heading west on I-80, passing through the Delaware Water Gap, and then trekking through Pennsylvania and Ohio before traveling north to Detroit. The hardest part was crossing Pennsylvania. It felt like an endurance test! The view was beautiful, but the sheer length of the state made me bone weary.

Though taking breaks at Pennsylvania rest stops was a must, I dreaded them. After a long run, I always imagined that we were farther across the state than we actually were. At each stop, a large map pinpointed our exact location. You know the kind of map I'm talking about. It usually has a big red arrow that says, "You are HERE." I never liked what that arrow told me. Wherever it said we were never matched where I hoped we would be.

I didn't celebrate those arrows because they brought me face-to-face with a reality I did not want to accept. If the arrow said we were halfway across Pennsylvania, I wanted to be three-quarters of the way across, and if it said we had traveled three-quarters of the state, I wanted to be in Ohio already. Obviously, the arrows were not the problem. They did not tell me what I wanted to hear, but they told me the truth about where I was.

There is a marketplace term for what the red "You are HERE" arrow reveals: It is called current reality. It is precisely where you are right now, and it is essential to the process of moving forward.

In analytical systems thinking, current reality addresses the root causes of organizational problems. Instead of using red arrows, organizations come to terms with where they are by creating current reality trees (CRTs). These diagrams help organizations' leaders and managers pinpoint their problems and identify any constraints that may be involved. Generally speaking, a constraint is anything that limits or restricts a person or entity from performing a particular action. It can make that person or entity feel unable to move forward and compelled to avoid the constraint at all costs.

You're probably wondering what that has to do with the negative thoughts and emotions associated with mental anguish. The connection is in how we deal with our current reality. My reaction to rest-stop signs was similar to my struggle with severe anxiety and depression. I saw both as impediments, and I had a hard time accepting their existence. Where I was and how long it took to go somewhere better seemed unacceptable. My current reality was not where I thought I should be.

Although the two situations were similar, one significant difference existed between them. The red arrows on the maps revealed an external reality. My "problem" was the state of Pennsylvania and how long it took to drive through it. My struggle with anxiety and despair was internal and was always with me. Though I could eventually drive out of Pennsylvania, I had no apparent way to leave the state of anxiety. Even the tiniest steps on that journey required every bit of strength I had.

During that dark season, two men whom I count as gifts in my life gave me much-needed care. One (my therapist) did so in a professional capacity, and the other (a dear friend) did so from a personal, scriptural, and pastoral perspective. Both were extremely competent therapeutically and offered sound counsel, and both were deeply committed to my well-being. Unfortunately, the last thing I wanted to hear from either of them was the one thing both kept saying—that I needed to accept my emotions and stop avoiding them.

It has been said that we are the sum total of everything we have ever thought, felt, said, and done. When caring people invited me to accept my struggle, I did not want to hear it, and I vehemently resisted. The sum total of everything I had ever thought, felt, said, and done would not let me. I had long conditioned myself to believe that I could summon my willpower and resist any constraining situation. I believed that if I rebuked it or paid it no mind it would have to go away. As the saying went in my spiritual tribe, "When in doubt, cast it out!"

Resisting Acceptance, Embracing Avoidance

The matter seemed simple: My suffering was demonic and had no business showing up in my life. Therefore, God would not allow or expect me to endure it, and it was my job to rebuke it. But every time I rebuked the thing, it seemed to turn around and rebuke me back. Nothing ever changed, and my suffering continued. Such realities were hard to deal with and even harder to reconcile.

Before my season of mental anguish, I remember watching Dr. Phil McGraw on television. As he interviewed his guests, I would help him psychoanalyze them. Often, I came up with the right answers regarding their troubles, which made me feel smart and capable—until I was in deep pain and couldn't psychoanalyze or heal myself.

I was never an "anti-psychology" type of preacher. I studied psychology because I believe the discipline has value. But I studied it with the Scriptures in mind. And yet spiritual warfare is also very real to me. So, in my suffering, the idea of rebuking my condition (with conviction, of course) seemed logical and even attractive. But when rebuking failed to work, I discovered the idea's flaws. What I thought I knew so well was being tested. I had prided myself in understanding the renewal of the mind. I prided myself in the testimonies of people around the world who received breakthroughs and deliverance from messages I preached. After all, the "breaker's anointing" was on my life and ministry, and I preached on breakthrough often.

Yet I could not navigate my perfect storm.

The answers I once trusted no longer seemed of any use. Absolutely nothing worked—*nothing*. It wasn't because everything I ever learned was wrong (although some of it was). It was because a red arrow was telling me where I was, and I refused to listen. Being a New York Italian who grew up singing Sinatra's "My Way"[1] probably didn't help me. Stubbornness seemed to be in my genes.

The two gifted men who walked me through that season would certainly attest to my resistance. Because I continued to recoil, I entered a prolonged period of internal resistance that was much more unconscious than I realized. Yet the finger of God would not let me run forever.

David prayed, "Search me, O God, and know my heart; test me and know my thoughts. See if there is any wicked [hurtful] way in me, and lead me in the way everlasting" (Psalm 139:23–25). Obviously, David understood that certain issues were escaping his conscious awareness and impeding his movement in God's intended direction. Those issues kept him from flourishing as God intended him to flourish. To move forward, David needed God to bring them out of the depths and up to the surface, so he could face and ultimately erase them.

Ironically, the renowned depth psychologist, Carl Jung, said something along those lines: "We cannot change anything until we accept it. Condemnation does not liberate, it oppresses."[2] Jung's words are not for other people who seem to have emotional problems. They are personal, and they are for us. There are things we need to accept, and that includes the negative emotions and thoughts we experience.

I certainly had to come to terms with mine. Condemning my pain did nothing but deepen the oppression that plagued my heart and mind. But changing course was not easy. I had no clue *how* to accept what I was going through. Looking back, I saw acceptance as a threat. Whatever was going on inside me was negative, so fighting it seemed best. Armed to the teeth theologically and psychologically, I fought for my life. I was sure I had the answers, and I was convinced I did not deserve the hell I was going through. I thought God would surely back me up.

Little did I know how good I was at getting in my own way! The harder I fought, the more defeated I became. It never occurred to me that my approach was prideful. I thought I was called to fight with everything I had. And because I believed my life hung in the balance, I saw my survival skills as being crucial.

From my perspective, fighting did not mean accepting my negative emotions and painful thoughts. That was out of the question. I wasn't Job! He was a good man who had some lessons to learn, and his situation was different from mine. Jesus came long after Job's day and shed light on human suffering. The redeemed are not called to suffer. Suffering is "Old Testament stuff."

Oh, how mixed up my thinking was—and how deftly the Spirit of God worked to reveal the truth! Considering all I knew about psychology, I knew little about the biases and filters that were blinding me. What the Spirit was asking of me was much different from what I *thought* He was asking. I thought *acceptance* was synonymous with *resignation*, but the words are worlds apart.

Distortions in my thinking were operating at an unconscious level and obscuring my path forward. God understood my needs and was offering to make a way out of no way. It was the very thing I longed for, *but I could not see it.*

Faulty Thinking Happens

A graduate degree in psychology does not guarantee protection against faulty ways of thinking. Every human being lives with cognitive distortion, which the *APA Dictionary of Psychology* defines as "faulty or inaccurate thinking, perception, or belief."[3] The APA adds, "An example [of cognitive distortion] is overgeneralization. Cognitive distortion is a normal psychological process that can occur in all people to a greater or lesser extent."[4]

These distortions typically escape our conscious awareness. Although we might detect them in other people, we rarely recognize them in ourselves. Until we see them, they are free to affect how we think. They come in many forms,[5] and all of them are common. For example, to overgeneralize is to see a single event in such an overarching way that you use it to interpret everything else in your life. Suppose you apply for a promotion at work but are turned down. If you overgeneralize the experience (which you might also perceive as a failure), you might assume you will be turned down for every future promotion you seek. Although you might not be consciously aware of the thought, it could influence your future behavior, causing you to adopt a *once a failure, always a failure* mentality that makes patterns of failure more likely.

To deal with faulty ways of thinking, you first need to recognize them. When you do, your avoidance strategies and other self-sabotaging habits lose their power. I'm not saying that your mindset will change overnight. No quick fixes exist for the process of growth, development, and maturity in Christ. These come from living a cross-shaped (or cruciform) life. You *can* inherit the promises, but doing so takes faith and patience, and that involves time.

While we are on this subject, let's address a common form of overgeneralization that exists in some churches. It is one I wrestled with during my dark season. The reason I felt called to fight my negative emotions and thoughts was the conviction that I wasn't wrestling with flesh and blood. The idea comes from Ephesians 6:12, which says that "our struggle is not against enemies of blood and flesh, but against the rulers, against the authorities, against the cosmic powers of this present darkness, against the spiritual forces of evil in the heavenly places."

Of course, the verse is 100 percent accurate, but I was only partly right in applying it to my situation. Some of what I experienced was demonic. That wasn't *the whole truth*, however. In fact, the demonic was the least of my problems. That might be hard to hear if you have been taught that every problem and pain comes from a spirit. I have certainly heard teachings along those lines, and I was taught that if I kept rebuking demonic spirits, they would quit attacking me, and my problems would be solved.

If that is what you were taught, it won't help you in the long run. For the record, the original apostles never taught that. Neither did the great fathers and mothers of the Church whom God used mightily from the Church's inception onward. Yet we teach this idea in popular Western culture, more out of habit and a lack of understanding than a genuine awareness of our rich Christian heritage.

When you read the writings of great voices in the ancient Church, what they teach can seem shocking. They spoke about the process of purification and cleansing. They focused on developing their spiritual senses so they could discern good and evil—not through attention-getting spiritual "dramatics," but with the quiet confidence that is grounded in maturity. Their writings are nothing like the quick-fix spirituality that poses as truth today. The two have almost nothing in common. Where the ancient teachings bring lasting freedom, the current approaches keep God's people chasing the wind. That is serious business! Teaching God's people to live in denial only leads them to wear "happy faces" while they languish. It does not resolve the real pain in their lives.

Later on in the book, I will take a deeper dive into cognitive distortions as I further describe my painful moments of facing an unwelcome current reality. For now, let me say that I get it. Because of the Fall we are afraid to admit our struggles. We imagine no one will accept us if we admit that our spiritual assumptions don't work. The dilemma reminds me of the Hans Christian Andersen story, "The Emperor's New Clothes." Deceitful weavers promised to create a special wardrobe for the emperor. All the clothing they "created" was imaginary. They went through the motions of dressing the emperor, but they left him stark naked! Because of his high position, no one dared say so except a young boy who did not fear the truth. He saw the fraud for what it was, and he spoke up!

Survival Mode and What-Ifs

Even when Andersen's fictitious emperor realized his nakedness, he continued the charade. In my season of suffering, I was a bit like him. Though I would eventually have to face the facts, for a time I tried to adapt and cope with the stress I experienced. That led to what medical science calls the fight-or-flight response, which is a physiological reaction to something mentally or physically frightening. Often, it is so taxing that we perceive it to be terrifying. I'm not suggesting it's not terrifying or traumatic. It might be both. In any case, the body and mind enter survival mode, ready to fight or take flight.

Consider this analogy: You discover a tiger is loose in your home. Within moments you experience an intense adrenaline rush, which is a natural response to danger. Your body and mind use that adrenaline to heighten your response to the crisis and focus your faculties on survival. One choice is to find a room with a door and shut yourself in. Behind that door, you feel safer, and your fight-or-flight response recedes. Eventually, your body returns to a normal, restful state.

But how would you respond if you were being pursued by an invisible creature, a menace you could not see or detect? You would have no way to know where it was or when it might show up. And closed doors would offer little or no protection. In that situation, you would remain on alert, stuck in survival mode with wave after wave of adrenaline rushing through your system for an indefinite period. Assuming it was not a man-eating menace, you would not fear bodily harm. But the presence of that menace would prey on your thoughts and torment you. The tiger might have picked your bones clean, but the invisible menace would eat away at your mind, hour by hour and day by day.

When the bus finally ran over me, I fought my symptoms, tackling them the way you would tackle a tiger running loose in your home. But my symptoms were not the real issue. I was facing an invisible menace that had fed on my stress responses *for years.* All that time, the menace fed my survival instincts, so that both the creature and my determination to fight it kept growing. Stalked by an invisible enemy, my heightened state of alarm continued in the form of unending what-ifs:

> *What if the invisible creature shows up when I'm in a meeting?*
> *What if it shows up when I'm alone?*
> *What if the menace appears when I'm working?*
> *What if it torments me when I'm at home with loved ones?*
> *What if that menace shows up when I'm conversing with So-and-So?*

The what-ifs can go on and on. *Merriam-Webster* defines them as "suppositional questions,"[6] which involve things that might happen. Though most of them will never happen, anxiety keeps them flooding your mind anyway. Your what-ifs are not about the tiger in the next room; they are about intangibles. They involve your expectations, how you see your world, and what your imagination says is in your future. They are not born from reasonable or genuine fears; they are driven by the anxiety that is rooted in previous traumas.

For the record, not every trauma involves profound violence or catastrophic loss. According to Matthew Tull, a psychology professor who specializes in post-traumatic stress disorder and anxiety disorders, trauma is "any type of distressing event or experience that can have an impact on a person's ability to cope and function,"[7] which means that everyone has experienced trauma. It may be the loss of a job, the death of a loved one, a divorce, the severing of a close relationship, an assault, abandonment, an accident, abuse (of any kind), a physical injury or natural disaster, or witnessing a violent crime.[8] Traumas leave imprints in the form of "intrusive thoughts and memories" or a state of heightened alert when no imminent danger is present.[9]

What-ifs are one way of coping with the traumas we have endured. Scripture is clear: We live in a fallen world. Therefore, we deal with many difficult issues. We see how good can be corrupted and become evil, and we become skilled at developing avoidance strategies and other coping mechanisms to mitigate our apprehensions. While these "tools" seem to help us in the short term, they exact a great cost over time.

When Help Feels Like Hurt

Earlier, I mentioned the competent and caring men who invited me to accept my anxiety and despair. They were right, but they were up against my well-honed, deeply embedded, cognitively distorted avoidance strategies, which kicked in and refused to back down. That left me in high gear all the time. Even sitting still required all the effort and concentration I could muster. Wherever I went, my anxiety and depression went with me. I felt as though I'd been locked in a fully sealed panic room with no way out.

My mental and physiological state had become so intolerable that I could not bear even to consider acceptance. Pain had so distorted my perceptions that I thought my helpers were asking me to resign myself to my awful condition. Inside myself, I heard them say, *This is your new normal. This is how it's going to be. Accept it.*

The thought of one more day of oppression seemed like more than I could tolerate. But a *lifetime* of mental and physiological anguish? That was unthinkable.

Of course, the people who cared for me were not suggesting anything of the sort. They were not inviting me to accept a life sentence; they were urging me to accept my feelings for what they were, not what I thought they should be. If I did that, I could commit to moving past them. I needed to acknowledge the facts on the ground, not endorse them.

In the years since that dark season ended, I have often wondered how much shorter it might have been had I not fought it so hard. As my therapist often reminded me, I had not arrived in the dark place overnight. My coping mechanisms took decades to develop. Then, when all hell broke loose, they seemed like my only option.

It is obvious now that I had other options but chose a poor one. Though it seemed to offer a payoff in the moment, there was a balloon payment on the back end. I learned the hard way that avoiding or denying my suffering only led to prolonged pain and despair. The better option is to face the pain up front for the sake of long-term pleasure later.

We cannot choose the right approach, however, until we consciously assess our available options. For me, that meant becoming aware of my avoidance strategies so I could change course. As skillful as I was at avoidance, I didn't realize I was using it. I was living on automatic pilot, responding reflexively to circumstances I believed I should not have to face.

Do you see the conundrum I was in? I could not acknowledge my avoidance strategies until I accepted my negative emotions and painful thoughts. I was not fully conscious of the choices I was making, yet they perpetuated my suffering. The more I relied on avoidance, the stronger my resistance and cognitive distortions became. It wasn't safe to exist in the world I was experiencing, and it wasn't safe to admit that I lived there. I was boxed in and terrified of saying, "I see that red arrow. I acknowledge that red arrow. I admit the truth of that red arrow. And I accept what that red arrow is telling me: 'I am HERE! I *am* HERE!'"

"Here" was not where I wanted to be. I wanted a quick way out of "here." The therapist offered anything but, saying, "You didn't get here overnight, Mark, and you won't get out overnight either."

His words were hard to swallow. I realized that I was in this thing for the long haul, and no amount of magical thinking would get me out. What I'd seen paraded as faith was nothing more than a spiritualized form of denial, an attempt to explain away the reality of Christian suffering. Yes! Christ died for us, but He never promised us pain-free lives. That unsound approach to Scripture could not lead me to health and wholeness. And it won't help you either. What it produces is a futile resistance to *being with* your pain.

It is no wonder that anxiety and depression stuck with me for three and a half years. I could not escape either by exerting my will or denying my condition. Using my "faith" that way was not faith at all because it was not based in the truth. It was a distortion further entangling me in negative emotions and thoughts fueled by past traumas and cognitive distortions. I was so enmeshed in my pain and sense of self that I could not tell where I ended and my thoughts and feelings began.

As a result, *acceptance* sounded like a dirty word. Whenever I heard it, I wanted to groan a deep, disgusted "Ugh!" The thought of it triggered a tirade inside me—a litany of resistance and defiance words that kept coming until I finally relented and said, "I accept where I am."

Precisely when that happened, I cannot say, but it likely occurred by early 2008. Once it did, my situation started to change.

I realized that anxiety and despair were not my biggest problems, and I admitted that my avoidance had brought me the most harm.

Embrace Your Red-Arrow Moment

Remember these words from David? "Where can I go from your spirit? Or where can I flee from your presence? If I ascend to heaven, you are there; if I make my bed in Sheol, you are there" (Psalm 139:7–8). I love how beautifully they express his consciousness of God's abiding presence. Yet, in my painful season, I somehow lost touch with the Spirit's abiding presence *with me*. Internally, I felt that God's omnipresence did not penetrate my current reality.

That might seem strange, because I believed what David said, and I trusted the experience he described. Intellectually and theologically, I knew I wasn't alone in my suffering. So what could explain the disconnect? Was I attempting to flee my reality in order to avoid issues the Spirit wanted me to address? Was I trying to "ascend to heaven" through willful determination? Did those attempts cause me to "make my bed in Sheol"?

By God's grace I eventually sorted out those questions, as you will see. But that could not happen until I accepted what my red arrow was telling me. I had to stop making my bed in hell. I had to release the desire to jump out of my own skin. I had to come to terms with where I was and what I was feeling. I had to arrive at a "rest stop," turn to the truth, cling to the Triune God, and confess, "I am *here*."

I claim no bragging rights about moving out of that season because I have none. But I can brag on God, who loved me in my worst moments. He never gave up on this stubborn Italian from New York, and He will never give up on you, no matter where your red arrow says you are. Trust Him in this, and let it be your first step toward acceptance.

QUESTIONS TO PONDER

» On a scale of 1–10, if 1 is hardly at all and 10 is perfectly, where are you when it comes to admitting "I am here"? In other words, how well can you admit your current reality?

» Even in admitting your current reality, might there be distortions in your thinking?

» If so, how will you come to recognize those distortions so you can deal with them?

3

The Grunt Work of Getting Whole

Beloved, do not be surprised at the fiery trial when it comes upon you to test you, as though something strange were happening to you. But rejoice insofar as you share Christ's sufferings, that you may also rejoice and be glad when his glory is revealed.

1 Peter 4:12–13 ESV

Accepting my reality was a huge step, a pivot point in the direction of healing. It was not the last step, but it allowed me to make other adjustments in my ways of perceiving and interpreting life. Day by day, I became more aware of the avoidance strategies I used in the hope of separating myself from my anxiety. In chapter 1, I mentioned my dual penchants for ruminating about my history and believing I "should not" suffer from anxiety because Jesus suffered in my place. Both strategies helped to distract me in the moment but gave my anxiety more power in the long run.

These and other perspectives governed my unconscious mind,[1] which in turn governed my response to pain. Awakening to them took some work. You might say it was *grunt work*—the sheer discipline of putting one foot in front of the other, over and over again. Personally, I hate grunt work. I don't know who coined the term, but the sound of it makes me want to grunt. And I did grunt—a lot!

Dealing with my habitual ways of observing and interpreting my world required me to become more self-aware. This not only meant looking inward, it meant looking back and acknowledging that I was raised in an environment of anxiety and worry. That might sound dysfunctional to you, but it was normal for me. My dad modeled anxiety and worry, and it pained me to see it. I loved him very much, and he loved me. He was a man of broken dreams and many fears. Without realizing it, he taught me to live in worry and fear.

Children learn a lot just by watching. They absorb what goes on in their family systems and discover years later that they are the people from whom they have come. Just as Adam passed the distortions of death and sin to all generations, each generation brings its brand of brokenness to the family tree. Whatever stays broken gets passed down to the next generation, and unless we deal with it, we pass it on again.

These issues can haunt us! Many Christians believe that we can resolve them in healing services where curses are removed. That sounds great, and I believe in healing services. But they rarely, if ever, heal decades of dysfunction. I have pastored long enough to see generational patterns persist in families. I know the children and their parents and grandparents, and I know that all of us—not some of us—need to be healed from the inside out.

That kind of healing is not an event but a lifelong process of becoming conformed to the image and likeness of Christ. As we follow Him, the Holy Spirit sets us apart and helps us to become fully human. This is how we glorify Christ. The fancy name for it is *sanctification*. It is less about following "do's and don'ts" and more about allowing Christ to be more fully revealed in and through us. This is what I mean when I say that sanctification is not an event. From the beginning of our days to the end of this life, God's perfect love is at work, casting out our fears and releasing "the fullness of him who fills all in all" (Ephesians 1:23 ESV; see also 1 John 4:18).

As I write these words, I can feel the resistance they will stir. We humans don't care for long, drawn-out solutions. That is why we look for quick fixes. When my therapist told me there was no quick way out of my suffering, I wanted to tell him off. It felt like he was heaping more pain on my pile. In retrospect, he saved me years of unnecessary anguish and confusion. Like him, my deepest desire is not to add to your pain but to offer the kind of hope that can keep you moving forward.

Yes, grunt work lies ahead, but it will pay off. Remember that you cannot accept what you continue to deny, and you cannot be healed of what you will not accept. You can face your troubles honestly. It's not easy at first. No one wants to admit they're afraid. Many people find coping strategies and claim they are afraid of nothing. The rest of us scratch our heads and wonder, *How can I become as fearless as they are?*

Beloved, they are not fearless. They are in denial.

All of us experience fear. In our brokenness, however, we learn to mask, suppress, and numb ourselves to it. This is not a sustainable approach but a façade—a *lie*. The more we suppress our fear, the more we feed it. The sooner we own it and stop deceiving ourselves, the sooner our healing can begin.

Facing the Fear with Truth

Dr. Karl Albrecht says that all humans experience five basic fears: "extinction" (death), "mutilation," "loss of autonomy," "separation" (including abandonment and rejection), and "ego-death" (such as humiliation and shame, and a sense of worthlessness).[2] Notice that death tops the list. It is, in fact, the grandaddy of the other four fears. We think of it as the fear of death itself. But it is also the fear of dying.

When we misunderstand what the Scriptures say about fear and faith, we are tempted to dismiss Dr. Albrecht's list. After almost five decades of helping people, I assure you that he is telling the truth. *We experience fear*, whether we are Christians or not. Why else would the command, "Fear not" or "Do not fear" appear throughout Scripture? (See Isaiah 41:10, 13, 14; Joel 2:21; Matthew 10:31; and John 12:15, for example.) We need to understand from a scriptural perspective how fear operates. That doesn't mean ignoring the data from psychology. Statistics do not refute Scripture; they simply confirm the universality of our fears.

If you don't want fear to rule you, don't let the powers of darkness know more about you than you know about yourself. When the bus hit me, my enemy knew more about my susceptibilities than I did. My ignorance was not blissful. It was miserable, and it put me at a disadvantage. When I felt the weakest, I had to climb out of that hole and find a new place of self-awareness. Talk about grunt work!

In retrospect, I was like those who claim to be fearless. I had unconsciously (and perhaps consciously) convinced myself that I was invincible. That is exactly what my dad had done. Although he was steeped in worry and anxiety, his manner said, *I've got my act together.* He was not a dishonest man. He was a man impaired by fear and working with any coping skills he could find. His façade seemed to work until his own dark season came at around age fifty. Ironically, my struggle started around the same age. It might appear that the devil attacked me the same way he attacked my dad but through a different set of fears. Even if that is partially true, it is an oversimplification—

the kind of explanation many people offered me at the time. Although they used Scripture to back up their words, their assumptions were not necessarily scriptural.

Let me explain what I mean. Those who offered pat answers to my struggle usually did it by proof-texting. Early in my educational journey, I learned a maxim that helps me stay on track: "A text without a context is a pretext for a proof text." There is a world of difference between using proof texts and "rightly handling the word of truth" (2 Timothy 2:15 ESV). Proof-texting is rampant, especially in Western culture. It is not faithful to Scripture because it singles out texts to justify (or prove) particular positions. In other words, it ignores context and misses the larger story that Scripture tells. People can even use it to justify ideas that are plainly unscriptural!

For example, Jesus and Paul both admonished us not to be anxious (see Matthew 6:25; Philippians 4:6). So when people become anxious, we extract those verses and say, "Quit being anxious." (Hopefully with more compassion than that!) We reduce the Scriptures to bromides and dispense them like candy. Instead of helping the people we care about, we forget to empathize or respect their cries for help. Our words become hollow because they misrepresent what Jesus and Paul taught.

Consider Jesus' suffering at Gethsemane, where He faced unimaginable anxiety and stress. How might we have responded to His agony? When He collapsed and great drops of blood burst through His pores, would we have told Him to "quit being anxious"? Would we have plucked a line from His Sermon on the Mount and dismissed His suffering? Do we believe even now that He should not have experienced the distress that the Gospels describe?

Paul's experiences raise similar questions. In his letters to the Corinthians, he admitted to being "in weakness, in fear, and in much trembling" (1 Corinthians 2:3 NKJV). The apostle Paul was no Marvel superhero. He was a human being who accepted his humanity and never pretended to be invincible. He freely shared his concerns for the church he planted, and he worried about their know-it-all mentality. Instead of hiding his emotions, he disclosed them. He did not succumb to worry; he simply told the truth and continued putting one foot in front of the other.

Paul was explicit about what he was up against. In 2 Corinthians 1, he minced no words:

> We do not want you to be unaware, brothers and sisters, of the affliction we experienced in Asia; for we were so utterly, unbearably crushed that we despaired of life itself. Indeed, we felt that we had received the sentence of death so that we would rely not on ourselves but on God who raises the dead.
>
> 2 Corinthians 1:8–9

Paul outright admitted that he despaired of life! In other words, he wasn't sure his life was worth living. His thoughts and emotions were so painful that he felt "unbearably crushed." He certainly seems to have accepted his reality. After all, he shared the details in writing. Later, in describing the profound opposition he faced in Macedonia, he wrote, "When we arrived in Macedonia, our bodies had no rest, but we were pressed from every direction—conflicts on the outside, fears within" (2 Corinthians 7:5 BSB).

"Conflicts on the outside, fears within." Have you been there? Do you hear the profound stress in Paul's words? Can you imagine cherry-picking what he wrote in Philippians 4:6 and telling him to "be anxious for nothing" (NKJV)? What a slap in the face that would be, and what an insensitive misapplication of his words!

There are real reasons why we short-circuit when we witness or experience pain. When Jesus agonized in the Garden, the three disciples He invited along were so overwhelmed by His suffering that they went to sleep. I believe they couldn't handle what they saw. We often feel the same way. We cannot handle the things we witness, and we long to escape the challenges we face. So we put on our "invincible" faces and hand out platitudes to the suffering—including ourselves.

Believe me, I understand the reflex. But shrinking back only keeps us captive. Facing our suffering and the suffering of others is part of our healing. The examples I just shared about Jesus and Paul helped me through my season of pain. Their suffering told me that mine had meaning! I realized that it was not random but was rooted in deep love and concern for the issues I faced. It was human pain, and no one escapes life without it. So I kept putting one foot in front of the other, and from time to time I grunted!

Identifying the Accuser's Voice

I love and respect the disciplines of theology and psychology and am still pursuing my education. What I have learned helps me to help others.

Strangely enough, I was less able to help myself. The accuser of the brethren pummeled me with the irony, quoting the proverb, "Physician, heal yourself!" (Luke 4:23 NKJV). His voice was unmistakable, but other voices chimed in. Even some dear preacher friends asked, "Why don't you just use your anointing to get rid of this thing?"

Beloved, if that isn't the voice of the accuser speaking through human lips, I don't know what is. At the time, I didn't have the emotional or volitional wherewithal to answer back, and probably for good reason. Somewhere within myself I agreed with them and believed I should have been able to "just get over it."

That is when I finally understood Job's terrible pain. Not only was it emotional, psychological, and physical, but it was insult added to injury! Job's friends doled out declarations and heaped fresh wounds upon him, claiming to speak for God.

Instead of holding their tongues and sitting with their friend, they judged him. Instead of comforting him, they served up blame. And instead of identifying and empathizing with him, they crushed his hope.

We often do the same. I'm not exactly sure what makes techniques and "how to's" so attractive in our culture, but we have turned the gospel into a menu of methods. We believe that using them in just the right way will open just the right doors. Like magic, our troubles will evaporate, and life will look the way we expect and want.

There is a certain amount of pride in that approach. We act as if we have all the answers, but we know far less than we realize. I never saw this Pharisaic tendency more clearly than I did during and since my dark season. That experience changed me! I read the Scriptures differently, I listen to people differently, and I minister to them differently. I'm not suggesting that everything I used to say or do was irrelevant or unhelpful. But I see more of the picture now. Though certain aspects of what I'm teaching today sound like what I taught for decades, I am now far more aware of how much I have yet to learn.

God used me when I thought I had it all together. He did it because He is merciful and gracious. And He did it for the sake of Jesus and those who suffer. It was also for my sake, so I could mature and fulfill His call on my life. Of course, the accuser never mentioned God's mercy. He only harped on my mess. But all the while, the Lord kept leading me into an open place. My role was to follow Him in the utter nakedness of my faith. I had to trust that He was in my darkness. I had to trust Him when I had no goose bumps to encourage me and no signs saying, *You will soon be out of the woods.* All of it was part of the grunt work of my deliverance.

If you feel overwhelmed by challenges that seem to come out of nowhere, you understand the nakedness of faith. The accuser will remind you day and night of how vulnerable you are. The fact is that whatever resources you have, whether they are plentiful or sparse, they are inadequate to set you free. My darkest season helped me realize this truth and come to terms with my dependency on God. The accuser is relentless, but so is our King.

Leaning on the Jesus in Others

The more I learn about the human psyche, the better I understand how the accuser works. And the more I look to Jesus, the better I understand how He "lifes me." When we experience trauma, the simple act of putting one foot in front of the other can seem impossible. It did to me, and I could not have made my way alone.

I've already mentioned the two precious men who walked me through the darkness, day by day. One is a friend who pastors in the Northeast. In my toughest moments, when I felt bereft of God's presence, the Jesus I saw in him gave me hope. When I could not find the words of faith within myself, I borrowed his words. I reminded myself of what he said, because I heard Jesus' voice in his voice.

Unless you have been somewhere like where I have been, this might sound peculiar, especially coming from someone who has preached Jesus all over the world. It was peculiar to me, too, but it taught me something paradoxical about trust. It's about the excruciating sense of absence you feel when you are suffering. Part of it is the seeming absence of the omnipresent God who cannot possibly be absent. There is also the absence of the inner "want to" that once propelled you forward. And there is the perceived absence of the Holy Spirit's encouragement, not because the Spirit has abandoned you, but because you cannot hear His sound.

Bear in mind that we are talking about grunt work, the work of moving forward when our world spins off its axis, and all seems lost. If you have ever tried to sink a spade into a barren, neglected patch of ground, you know what grunt work is. That hard soil will vehemently resist your effort to penetrate it. If you want to make the land fruitful and beautiful again, you will sink that spade over and over again, no matter the effort. Your motivation will keep you working until the soil is ready for seed.

But during periods of sustained suffering, your "want to" disappears. The devil swears you are finished, and you fear that God and His Spirit have left you to your own devices. The paradox is that your sense of absence can drive you to a renewed trust in the presence that *never* leaves you. In the barren places, the ministrations of God's Word and staff comfort you. When life's liminal spaces stretch and exhaust your capacity and will, God works through the people who are committed to walking with you. He uses their experience and perspectives to remind you of what is true. He teaches you to appropriate from them whatever might apply in your dark season.

During my protracted struggle, my friend's voice helped me to follow God when my inner witness and inner voice seemed to leave my temple. My sense of perspective disappeared, yet God kept leading me. He did it in the presence of reliable others who reminded me that I was progressing even when I saw no renewal in my routine and no revelation in my rituals. They helped me realize that although my progress was incremental, it was progress all the same.

Becoming Fully Human

The process of healing is tied to becoming fully human. Depth psychologist Dr. David Benner says that "the boundaries of the soul are difficult to delineate."[3] Benner's perspective draws on his understanding of psychology and theology. There is the keen awareness that humans are complex, with brokenness and beauty coexisting in everyone.

To become fully human, we need to understand that we live in language, emotions, feelings, and moods. These domains communicate continually, often without our conscious awareness. We are prone to drifting and living on autopilot. Particularly when we are under pressure, we can slip from the state of cogent, conscious awareness and let unconscious drivers (like avoidance strategies) take over. It is as though we are fast asleep behind the steering wheel of life. I can almost hear Paul saying, "Sleeper, awake! Rise from the dead, and Christ will shine on you" (Ephesians 5:14).

Awake indeed! To become human is to embark on more than a lifelong journey. We are continually in process, but until we receive our resurrected bodies at the consummation of the ages, the fullness of our humanity is incomplete. For now, our bodies are subject to decay and corruption because of Adam's sin. That doesn't mean our bodies are evil, as Plato believed and as gnostic heretics taught. They saw all matter as evil and believed that the goal of human existence is to escape matter altogether and become like angels. For Plato, only death could free us from our mortal bodies.

Sadly, some Christians sound a lot like Plato. The human body is not evil, however. If it were, why would God have created us this way? Why didn't He make us like angels or some other incorporeal beings? And why would Jesus take on an evil human body? Was His incarnation a colossal error?

I realize this subject is worthy of a book all by itself, but let this one point be clear in your mind: By divine design, we are embodied spirits. We are not "good" spirits trapped in "evil" bodies. Of course, in a fallen world, our bodies take a beating. Environmental, emotional, economic, social, and other stressors take a toll. Disease and calamity cause physical harm. Our bodies require continued care, but in our ignorance we often abuse them, largely by driving ourselves to achieve and succeed regardless of the cost. Trust me: The cost is exorbitant, and living that way will eventually bite you back.

I didn't learn that lesson from a book. I learned it the hard way. Part of the grunt work that began after I accepted my situation involved learning how not to burn the candle at both ends. I had lived that way too long and ignored the warning signals my body gave me. I paid little heed to my sleep deprivation and my increasing stress levels. Between my love and concern for loved ones and my local church family, I overextended myself. My commitment to the call of God has always been strong, but after the bus hit me, I learned to temper it with wisdom and some common sense.

When the drive for success is coupled with free-floating anxiety, a rude awakening is inevitable. Setting yourself up that way reveals a lack of self-awareness that always travels with a lack of others-awareness. Simply put, it indicates that your emotional intelligence is lagging. In that condition, almost anything can get the best of you. You tend to ignore what is worthy of your attention, and you conveniently compartmentalize your life. Instead of being an observer first, you become a reactor. And if anxiety happens to be your default reaction—watch out for the bus!

The journey to healing begins with acceptance, but the work that follows includes becoming fully awake and aware of what we are experiencing and admitting. Until we commit to this level of consciousness, we will never understand why we see and interpret life the way we do. Instead of taking ownership and living consciously from the inside out, we will continue to master avoidance strategies. In other words, we will live on autopilot.

If you can relate to what I am saying, do not condemn yourself. We are all guilty. Discarding avoidance strategies is part of the healing process, and coming off autopilot requires vigilance. The grunt work is simple but not always easy. Avoidance is a habit we develop to help us cope. Once we recognize it, we can break it. Then our ways of observing and interpreting life can be renewed, and we can live as we were created to live—from the inside out.

Beloved, the work of becoming whole might make you grunt, but it is worth it. I *promise*!

QUESTIONS TO PONDER

» Take an inventory of your life and what you have been taught. Ask yourself honestly if you thought the goal of your life was to be a "good Christian, then die and go to heaven." If you did, what might you be avoiding in your day-to-day life, and how is it robbing you of the power of the endless life of Christ right now?

» On a scale of 1–10, if 1 is total failure and 10 is total success (however you define them), where do you rate yourself and why?

» Does that rating stir up anything at an emotional level? What are those emotions telling you?

» If you respond negatively to your rating process, what negative feelings show up in your body as stress? How do you cope with them? In what ways is your coping ineffective?

4

Nothing's Perfect

Imperfections are not inadequacies; they are reminders that we're all in this together.

Brené Brown, *The Gifts of Imperfection*

Accepting what you cannot conquer immediately is not enough. You need to live with enthusiasm for the future. As someone once said, "Success is the ability to go from failure to failure without the loss of enthusiasm." During the hardest season of my life, however, I found it difficult even to come to the beginning of acceptance, and moving from acceptance to transformation proved far more challenging than I cared to admit.

You see, I had a deeply ingrained drive toward perfection. It was instilled from my earliest years by my dad's determination to keep me from failing as he thought he had failed. So driven, I was always striving to meet an impossible standard, reaching for a level of "success" I could not possibly touch because it wasn't real in the first place.

I cannot blame my dad for all of that. When I was very young, I somehow adopted the perfectionist framework. By the time I realized it, a core insecurity had already grown large inside of me. It told me I was not good enough, not smart enough, not talented enough. Like a gigantic octopus, its tentacles slowly choked me, crushing my heart and my hopes. I tried to live from the inside out. But I never really freed myself from the delusion that I could and should be perfect. I struggled against that monster deep into my journey and long after I thought I had bested it.

It might seem obvious, but in our circles it still needs to be said that healing does not always happen with the wave of a hand. In fact, the healing process often, if not always, makes us feel worse before it makes us feel better. It was painful for me to admit that I was dealing with anxiety and depression. And it was even more painful to accept that I could not fix myself or speed up the healing process, no matter how hard I tried. Once I came to terms with those realities, I began to discover how deep-seated certain negative beliefs and assumptions were in me, beliefs and assumptions that needed to be removed. That was painful, too. But I was finally seeing myself clearly, and I was grateful for that.

Sooner or later, we must face our issues squarely. We cannot do that without self-awareness. Organizational psychologist Tasha Eurich's research focuses on two aspects of self-awareness.[1] She refers to the first and most basic aspect as internal self-awareness, which, as she explains, involves the ability to recognize what we value at our core—our dreams, our drives, what makes us tick. This aspect of self-awareness determines how we relate to the environment we live in and how we interact with others in that environment. Coming to that self-awareness is a costly process.

Human beings are meaning-makers by nature and by necessity. We are always "reading" our reality, always making sense of what is transpiring in and around us, although we often forget that we're doing it. You might say we are walking, talking sets of interpretations. How we see is inextricably bound up with who we are. So the cognitions and perceptions that lead to our interpretations of reality inevitably reveal *and* form our characters.

Once I was ready to accept that I was suffering from anxiety and depression, I thought I had essentially beaten it. I assumed that mere awareness of the problem was sufficient. Yet we are complex creatures, and the world can be a difficult place. Healing is a process that takes time and can be convoluted. Living from the inside out isn't nearly as easy as the self-help gurus suggest.

I am introspective and analytical. My mind can work for me, and when it does, life can be wonderful. My mind can also work against me, however. Precisely because I'm inner-directed and thoughtful, I weigh everything. Doing this under the pressure of needing to be perfect and needing not to fail becomes profoundly negative, leading to inflexibility and all kinds of ugly, aching feelings. As a result, my healing process took a long time, not because I was failing to do my part, but because I was the one who needed healing in so many ways. My healing process was painful, not because I failed, but because the pains in me needed to be worked out, which is painful all by itself.

The Feeling That Something's Missing

Most kids love to play in the snow. I was no different. And thankfully, as a child growing up in New York City, we had many icy, snowy winters. I have many fond memories of building snowmen and having snowball fights with my friends and family. But because it was so much fun, I made the same mistake

75

repeatedly: In my rush to get outside, I would grab my woolen mittens instead of the leather gloves my mom and grandma lovingly placed in my dresser drawer.

Wool was no match for wet snow and the bitter cold. But the exciting sounds of my cousins laughing and playing in the backyard made me feel that I was missing out on something too good to wait on. That feeling caused me to make foolish choices. Once I got outside, my hands would quickly freeze. But even then, I was having too much fun to care . . . until my hands got so cold that I couldn't move them or even feel them anymore. At that point, I would panic.

The *I'm missing something* feeling, rooted in hidden, un-resolved fears, proved to be a crucial part of the pain I endured in my dark season. In moving through that darkness, I learned a hard lesson: If the feeling of "missing something" makes us afraid, and if we never bother to work through why, that fear will eventually turn into worry and then anxiety. Once that anxiety takes hold in our unconscious, it dictates much of our lives.

That unconscious anxiety expresses itself in the toxic "What if?" questions I mentioned earlier, which slowly poison our cog-nition and perception.

From the time I was little, my dad wanted to make sure I didn't miss my opportunities the way he felt he had missed his. He therefore unconsciously and unknowingly seeded me with fear that would become anxiety. And when that anxiety mixed with my drive to be perfect, it became a lethal cocktail for the development of free-floating anxiety.

Micah Abraham explained that the adjective *free-floating* means that anxiety is present even when we aren't in danger.

When your fear is so persistent, distressing and disproportion-ate to the threat you're facing—sometimes even occurring in the absence of any real observable threat—this is when an anxiety disorder might be considered. If you're experiencing anxiety when no dangers are present, and it seems to occur without anything triggering it, you may have what we call "free-floating anxiety."[2]

Every time I felt I was "missing something," fear would grip me, and I would get caught in endless what-if cycles: "What if I mishandled that situation? What if I drop the ball on a family matter, or misread a need in the church? What will the consequences be?" My most haunting question—the one that supercharged my anxiety—was "What if this is my new normal, and what if it never changes?"

All of this "what-iffing" worsened dramatically when I hit my unexpected season of darkness. I encountered several crisis events, all of which happened in rapid succession. I cannot disclose them in detail because the worst of them involved close family members. I can, however, say that what happened took my fears over the edge. Under those circumstances, free-floating anxiety nearly suffocated me. The powers of darkness used my fear of "missing something" to afflict me at the core of my being.

Despite it all, God was with me, working in me below the level of my conscious awareness. I was not simply at the mercy of what was happening. I was in the mercy of God. He was doing for my tormented soul what my mom and grandma did for my freezing hands. That story replayed itself many times because I failed to stop and find the right gloves, and I failed to pay attention to the growing numbness of my hands. Panic would ultimately set in, and I would run inside, crying for my mom or my grandmother, knowing they could and would "fix it."

Notice, I put "fix it" in scare quotes. Our language so often reveals our erroneous views. In this case, "fix it" betrays our technical, mechanical thinking. We fix machines, not human beings! Yet we *are* human beings, forgiven sinners with a certain brokenness we cannot remedy. We don't need to be "fixed." We need to be healed and made whole.

In my moments of panic, Mom and Grandma always rushed to my aid and knew what to do. They removed my mittens and turned on the faucet, running hot water over my hands. Not hot to the point of scalding, but hot enough to remedy the issue. At first, my nearly frostbitten hands couldn't feel a thing. But soon they started to ache, and I began to cry. They held my hands under the water until the circulation returned, the color of my hands went from gray-white to pinkish red, and I could move my fingers again.

Accepting that my hands were frozen was not enough. It was just the beginning. My hands had to stay under the hot water, which meant things got worse before they got better. Similarly, the journey from the "frozenness" of my rigid and inflexible beliefs to the "thawing out" of fear's icy grip was excruciating. The journey to self-awareness is painful for all of us. That should not be surprising, because, as Carl Jung stated, "The most terrifying thing is to accept oneself completely." So let me say to you what I needed to hear myself: Do not be afraid! Tell God everything you fear to acknowledge. He cannot heal what you conceal, but He will heal everything you reveal.

I had to feel the pain in the healing process, as we all do. I had to face my deepest-rooted fear and embrace my imperfection. And I had to bring it all to speech before God—again and again and again. My fears ran deep, and breaking free from the monster's tentacles was anything but easy. For endless hours, days, weeks, even months, I struggled. The pain of doubting myself and fearing that I was irrelevant haunted me. I was face-to-face in the dark with a profound sense of failure. My prayers and petitions seemed useless. Time and time again, I worked to unburden myself of the deep-seated fear that was largely responsible for my anxiety and its eventual constant companion, despair.

I could offer a long list of books on emotional intelligence and self-awareness from brilliant social scientists, all of which deserve to be read. As we end this chapter, however, I want to share with you an ancient poem, written by one of the greatest doctors of the Church, Saint Augustine. Remarkably, the poem reveals the journey to self-awareness in relationship to Christ. Before I share it, let me encourage you to stop trying to fix yourself. You are not a machine. You are an embodied soul, a human being, totally unified from the inside out. You are not made up of mechanical parts, and you do not need a technician or mechanic. You don't need fixing or a fixer. Nor are you called to be perfect. You simply need healing, and Christ is your Healer. Let Him hold your hands under the water.

In that spirit of surrender, you can pray Saint Augustine's prayer as your own. I encourage you to do it often. I have learned in this season that praying prayers that were written long ago and handed down as part of the Great Tradition can be a very present help from the Holy Spirit in times of dire need. Bring these words to your lips often and ask the Holy Spirit to cause you to realize that this is part of the journey to self-awareness, a journey that leads to the healing in which you become all God means for you to be.

> Lord Jesus, let me know myself and know You,
> And desire nothing save only You.
> Let me hate myself and love You.
> Let me do everything for the sake of You.
> Let me humble myself and exalt You.
> Let me think of nothing except You.
> Let me die to myself and live in You.
> Let me accept whatever happens as from You.
> Let me banish self and follow You,
> And ever desire to follow You.
> Let me fly from myself and take refuge in You,
> That I may deserve to be defended by You.

Let me fear for myself, let me fear You,
And let me be among those who are chosen by You.
Let me distrust myself and put my trust in You.
Let me be willing to obey for the sake of You.
Let me cling to nothing save only to You,
And let me be poor because of You.
Look upon me, that I may love You.
Call me that I may see You,
And for ever enjoy You.
Amen.[3]

QUESTIONS TO PONDER

» Honestly ask yourself: Have I built my entire belief system in relation to faith or magical thinking? Do I believe that if I quote a Bible verse enough times, my problem will go away?

» Where are the emotional pains and difficult thoughts and feelings in your heart and mind that have not responded to that kind of thinking?

» Would you own those right now in the presence of God? Will you write them down and bring them to speech before Him?

5

Perplexity, Apprehension, Anxiety

The most confused we ever get is when we're trying to convince our heads of something our heart knows is a lie.

Karen Marie Moning, *Faefever*

Why are some thoughts and feelings more painful than others? It's because there's a difference between the ones you have and the ones that have you. If you have thoughts, you can sort through them easily enough. But if thoughts have you, they become impossible to manage.

To "thaw out" and get free of the thoughts and feelings that had me, I had to become more truly and fully self-aware and willing to change my timeworn evaluations of my past and my present. That meant questioning my beliefs and assumptions and comparing them to scriptural truth. I had to evaluate their origins: Were they Christ-centered, cross-shaped realities?

Or were they man's consumer-oriented, formula-driven techniques? Human techniques could not face evil squarely and reckon with its menacing presence. They could not affirm that the God of all comfort knew and loved me, profoundly and deeply. These questions were crucial. I had to become conscious of what my beliefs implied, and if I was flying blindly on autopilot, I needed to know it.

For too long I had so identified with certain negative evaluations of my experiences that I couldn't separate myself from them. Mind you, I had taught thousands of people about developing a nonjudgmental approach to life and accepting people, places, and events as they unfolded. I knew, at least intellectually, that learning to accept things as they were was part of knowing how to live the abundant life. I could teach and instruct others, but when I was the one standing in need of prayer, I entered unfamiliar territory. I already knew the truth as a mentor, leader, and pastor. But I did not know it *personally, for myself.*

When you are the one suffering serial restlessness and disease, when pain, numbness, and ache are your constant companions, it is nearly impossible to be objective. And when you lose your objectivity, you lose self-awareness—the ability to perceive yourself in a way that promotes health and well-being. You find yourself destabilized. Negative mantras well up in your self-talk. In my darkness, I had to learn to resist the voice that insisted: *This is the worst thing that could ever happen in my life!*

In the opening chapters of Genesis, when God placed man in paradise, his first charge was to name all the beasts of the field as God brought them before him. Whatever Adam named them, that is what they became. This was a prophetic and priestly function. God empowered man to bring things to speech, to speak words that would invoke and evoke the very identity and purpose of every beast of the field. This was about much more than the naming of animals. This was the power by speech to invoke meaning and destiny in the lives of these creatures.

As human beings, we are continually and simultaneously *being* and *becoming*. You might say that, at any given moment, half of who we are is the sum of everything we have thought, felt, said, and spoken from the days of our earliest existence. These dynamics involve our observations, which determine our interpretations. In other words, how we see dictates how we respond. Start paying attention to *how you see* what you are observing.

Remember, however, that time never stands still. It keeps moving forward. And that means we are never settled. We experience time as past, present, and future. So when life becomes difficult, what we bring to speech necessarily touches all three. How we define, name, and invoke what passes before us is crucial to what we experience from the inside out. If I name something This-Is-the-Worst-Thing-That-Could-Happen, I invoke a sense of foreboding, unrest, and uncertainty that continues as I move into the future. By verbalizing my interpretation of what I see unfolding, I bend my reality into an imprisoning place.

The Bible tells us that whatever Adam named a creature, that is what the creature became. If that was true for Adam, doesn't it stand to reason that whatever I name will become what I name it? Trust me when I tell you that when I saw situations as "the worst thing that could have happened" in my life, I believed it. As I explained earlier, I can't share all the painful realities of that season, but they really felt like the worst things that could happen. It was virtually impossible not to see them that way. The weight was oppressive, and the tension produced was hellish. The toll on my mind and my body was devastating.

What Does Dante's *Inferno* Have to Say to Me?

Dante's *Inferno* begins with these words:

> In the middle of the journey of our life, I came to myself, in a dark wood, where the direct way was lost. It is a hard thing

to speak of, how wild, harsh and impenetrable that wood was, so that thinking of it recreates the fear. It is scarcely less bitter than death: but, in order to tell of the good that I found there, I must tell of the other things I saw there.[1]

Growing up, I heard a great deal about midlife crises. I also remember having to read and write about them in some of my undergraduate psychology classes. Reading and writing about a subject is theoretical. Living it is another matter. And here is one thing they never tell you in class: The middle of your life's journey might not arrive at the specific birthday you have in mind. Most of my friends who talked of midlife crises had theirs in their late thirties and early forties, but the "middle" of my journey came just past the half-century mark. I was all set to enter my fifties with confidence that I was in the prime of life. But instead of being at the point where everything "should be" coming together, my midpoint came in a dark wood where my own "inferno" threatened to swallow me whole.

Where I am is tied to *who* I am. Who I am is the sum total of all I've experienced and am experiencing. That encompasses my past and my present, but not my future. The future is about my *becoming*, not my being. By default, then, if I change nothing in the way I see reality, I will repeat the known past and carry it with me into the unknown future.

Yet I am more than the total of my thought processes, feelings, and actions. And I have been blessed with the powers of imagination and intuition. My imagination can envision what is *and* what can be. And my intuition can grasp what is real despite what seems to be true. Thus, it is possible for *what I can be* to be greater than *what I have been*. So if I am continuously being and becoming, then half of who I am is the sum total of all those realities, and the other half—the half that is tied to becoming—is rooted in what I can imagine for myself and of myself.

The future is shaped by the choices we make in the present moment. But no choice is more important than the choice about how we see ourselves and our experiences. If (based on my entanglement with ugly thoughts about myself and my experiences) I choose to see the past and the present in the worst possible light, then the future will remain dark. If I convince myself that things will only get worse, I will find it impossible to think, feel, or act hopefully, faithfully, or lovingly. It becomes impossible to change. If my imagination is imprisoned in worst-case scenarios, driven by anxiety, trapped in endless cycles of *what-if* thinking, I will remain locked in an inferno of my own making.

When "the worst thing that could ever happen" happened, it wasn't just one bad thing. It felt as though all hell broke loose on my life. I would not equate my suffering and loss with Job's, but I do know what it is like to sit in the ashes and scrape the "boils." I know about the place of vexation and deep anguish—and I so wanted to escape the pain. Believe me, I was angry—with myself, with others, and even with God. I felt He had let me down—and I wasn't let down easily.

I hit bottom, and I hit it really, *really* hard. I became one with all my judgments and was no longer acceptable to myself. Imagine having to face the dark wood in the middle of life's journey, only to discover that it is the terrain of your own inner being. Saint Augustine found that out, and so did I.

During one of my darkest moments, I had a profound dream. A persistent knot in my stomach had kept me awake nearly all night. When I finally dozed off, the knot remained. My dream began in my paternal grandparents' house, where I grew up from the time I was about three years old. I experienced so much comfort in that house. Grandma and Grandpa lived downstairs, and so did various uncles, aunts, and cousins. Though I was an only child, I was never without the companionship and care of my family.

I felt safe in that home. I felt secure. I felt loved. No, nothing was perfect. We had our family pains. We had our sorrows. We had dysfunctions. But we also had a lot of love there. As I matured, that house became part of my internal environment. I aspired to embody all that that house represented for me, so to dream about it was not a big surprise. But what happened in the dream *did* surprise me.

Over the course of my advanced studies, I have done much research on dreams and dreaming. I am familiar with the landscape of dreams, and I have learned how the unconscious speaks to us through everyday metaphors and symbols. Still, those studies did not and could not prepare me for the lived experience of this dream.

In the dream, I went down the stairs into the basement, which had a large family dining table on one side, a kitchen table in the middle, stoves and an industrial sink, a pantry, and a little spare bedroom under the stairs. A sheet hung over the doorway to the back of the basement where the old furnace stood, along with some things that Grandpa kept stored. As kids, we avoided that part of the basement. The lighting was poor, and our imaginations ran wild in the dark. The shadows made us feel as though ghosts and goblins waited there to consume us.

In the dream, I stood face-to-face with the sheet that hung in front of that doorway. I knew it was dark on the other side. I also knew I had to go back there. Something I had to see beckoned me. The knot in my stomach was very present during my dream. As I prepared to pull back the sheet, that knot sent shockwaves from the center of my being to the farthest extremities of my limbs. Though I was asleep, I could feel the shockwaves in my body. It was painful.

I stepped into the dark. The concrete ended at the doorway, and after the first step, I felt my feet on the dirt floor I knew from my childhood. I saw the furnace way in the back to my left. The storage shelves where Grandma kept all her canned tomatoes and fruit were far in the back, ahead of me. I spotted my grandfather's tools in their cubbyhole, which was broken into the wall that supported the front of the house.

I knew I had to go toward the far wall on my right. Normally, that was where the concrete wall on the right side of the house met a Sheetrock wall to the right of the doorway. But as I moved toward the corner, another doorway appeared, one that didn't exist in real life. Another sheet hung over the second doorway, and I vividly remember being afraid to pull back that sheet. Nevertheless, I knew I had to do it.

When I did, I found myself standing in a dark cemetery in the dead of winter. The trees were barren, and dead leaves were strewn across the grounds. Dark limbs and branches hung low and were reaching everywhere. I felt like I was in a horror flick. In the dead center of the cemetery stood a gravestone—an ancient, granite Celtic cross. It was weatherworn and had been there for centuries, standing half uprooted above the grave it marked. Somehow, as I stood apprehensive and anxious, that gravestone conveyed profound significance to me. At the time, I had no idea what it meant. As I'll share with you later, its meaning became clear only at the end of my dark season. Yet in that moment, I was perplexed and very uneasy. Just then, when I became fully aware of my perplexity, apprehension, and anxiety, I awakened.

In that moment, I knew that triad—perplexity, apprehension, and anxiety—was the threefold emotional knot that would not let go of my stomach or my life. And I knew that those three intertwined realities required fresh observation and new interpretation so I could get free from them. I recognized that they were fruits, and they sprang from roots I needed to sever. You might say I knew in my knower (even while I was resistant to saying it out loud) that the inner work I needed to do required taking that knot in hand and learning to untie it.

Once untethered from the knot, I could move freely into the future God hoped for me. I could have thoughts without my thoughts having me. I could rest in the idea that I was both *being* and *becoming* day by day, not through self-effort but by grace, and in God's own timing.

This is what God offers us in every moment. With confidence, I can tell you that taking Him up on His "offers" always leads to healing—the healing you and I want and need.

QUESTIONS TO PONDER

» Look at what pains you emotionally and psychologically. Then consider the thoughts that accompany all of that. Can you identify your self-talk?

» Get in touch with that self-talk and write it down on paper so you can look at it objectively. When you write it down and read it, what do you notice?

» Where are those perceptions of that pain taking you in terms of the outcomes you are experiencing emotionally and psychologically? How are they impacting you physically?

6

Soul and Body

What does your anxiety do? It does not empty to-morrow, brother, of its sorrows; but, ah! it empties to-day of its strength.

Alexander McLaren, "Anxious Care"

With McLaren's words in mind, I want to take a slight detour in my story, right in the middle of telling you how I learned to untie the threefold knot of perplexity, apprehension, and anxiety. This is an essential detour, I believe, because so many of us have forgotten that we are embodied souls.

Somewhere in our awareness we recognize that we are profoundly fragmented and in need of healing. The ancient doctors of the Church saw sin as a disease from which we needed to be healed by the love of Jesus. When the Fall occurred, the result was the profound fragmentation of our internal beings and the fracturing of the relationships external to us, including our relationships with God, neighbor, creation, and purpose.

Through the Spirit's sanctifying power, the work of the cross heals our fragmentation. But that work takes time. Over the long course of our lives, we move ever closer to the fullness and shalom that God has promised. But if we are truly self-aware, we know that no matter how far we progress in our journey with Jesus, we always have further to go. No matter what we've done, we still have unfinished business to address. Even if the work in Christ is finished, we still have to ask for our "daily bread."

One of the deepest signs of our fragmentation is the split we experience between our minds and our bodies. We've all heard talk about the gap between our heads and our hearts, and in future chapters we'll address that problem as a necessary part of the healing journey. For now, however, let's consider why Western Christians tend to live out their Christianity in their heads, often ignoring what's going on in their bodies—as if our bodies are totally separate from who we are as persons.

As I said at the beginning, many of us forget that we are embodied souls or embodied spirits. God created us to be embodied. This was the understanding of the ancient Church, all the way back to the days of Jesus. This is also what the ancient Jewish faith taught—the faith that Jesus learned from His teachers. But for some reason, contemporary Christians in the Western world often ignore what's going on in their bodies, or they pay the wrong kind of attention to it.

So often preachers find ways to devalue human feelings. I have heard countless sermons on the insignificance of feelings. No doubt you've heard them, too. In addition, many preachers confuse emotions and feelings, leaving the impression that they are identical and indistinguishable. But they are not.

What Makes a Feeling a Feeling

What makes a feeling a feeling is that we feel it! Don't miss what I just said. It might not sound deep, and it is so obvious that we miss its profundity. Here's the point: We feel in our bodies! To know what I am feeling requires acknowledging that something is registering somewhere in my body.

Sermons that warn us against trusting our feelings encourage us to dismiss our feelings as irrelevant. But not listening to our bodies means dismissing one of the truth's most trustworthy witnesses. Often, our bodies try to tell us how stressed we are, how overworked we are, how frustrated we are, how angry we are, how burned out we are, and how tired we are. To ignore those messages is to ignore the voice of the truth—the voice of the Spirit that calls us toward life.

Tragically, we've been taught to treat our bodies as machines. If we have been raised in and formed by Christian subcultures that denigrate the body and delegitimize feelings, we're liable to distrust and abuse our bodies, even if we appear to be concerned about our "health." We might go to the gym, take vitamins, and watch our diet—all of which is well and good, of course—but that does not mean we know how to respect our body's truth. No matter how much we exercise, no matter how well we eat, if we delegitimize our feelings, we will lose touch with reality. In short, the failure to pay attention to the body's feelings is a surefire way to set ourselves up for a catastrophe.

I know this because I lived it. For years, I burned the candle at both ends. I was in high demand and was convinced that the work of the gospel required endless sacrifices of my time and body. I worked out. I ate well. I took tons of vitamins. I even prided myself self-righteously on the fact that I took no medications. Yet I continually ignored my body's warnings. Instead of heeding my stress levels and acknowledging my worry, restlessness, and feelings of overwhelm, I neglected sleep, failed to make time for rest, and resisted creativity and play. The work of the ministry demanded utter urgency, I thought, so I had no time for Sabbath. Mix that foolishness into the perfect storm that arrived in the middle of my life, and you have a recipe for a disaster!

As perhaps you already know, when you're running on adrenaline it's easy to numb out and lose touch with how exhausted you are. And when you've depleted your resources but continue to think that your "strong will" (something no one really has) will keep you moving forward safely, you will dismiss your body's warning signs until it is too late.

My body had been trying to tell me to slow down, take a break, take it easy, and get some rest. I needed to establish better sleep patterns, to disconnect from the pressures and problems that go with intense pastoral care and itinerant ministry. But I paid no mind to what my body was saying. You could describe my life at that time as "eat and run." I prayed, certainly. But I prayed "on the run." I studied, certainly. But I studied "on the run." The endless chatter of ministry demands played loudly on a loop in the back of my mind, even while I was praying and studying the Scriptures.

When I was supposed to be present in our family time, the chatter grew even louder. It became harder and harder just to "be there." In many ways, I lived in my head, detached and cut off from my body. From a psychological perspective, I knew the significance of the emotions that register in the mind, the feelings that register in the body, and the moods that pervade our overall attitude, but I mostly ignored what I knew. Why? Perhaps at some level I thought I was immune or bulletproof. Regardless, I found out that I wasn't, and I wasn't as self-aware as I thought. How dangerous. How foolish. How utterly tragic! And my case was anything but unusual.

If you've heard teaching on the renewal of the mind, you know the message usually begins with Romans 12:2: "Do not be conformed to this world, but be transformed by the renewing of your minds." Isn't it strange that we leap past the verse that comes before that? In Romans 12:1, Paul begs his readers to listen: "I appeal to you therefore, brothers and sisters, by the mercies of God, to present your bodies as a living sacrifice, holy and acceptable to God, which is your spiritual worship." Take a careful look at Paul's words. He is appealing to his listeners based on God's mercy. Do a careful study of mercy from a scriptural perspective and you soon discover it is tied to our need for forgiveness and healing.

So Paul is urging his brothers and sisters in Rome to come to terms with how broken they are, and he does this by nudging them first to pay attention to how they are living *in their bodies*. Here's the question, then: If Paul's appeal for mercy is predicated first and foremost on what the Roman Christians do with their bodies, so that through the offering of their bodies their minds might be renewed, isn't it obvious that I need to heed what my body is saying? If our bodies are temples housing the sacred presence of the Lord of glory, if we are one spirit with Him, then being mindful of and taking care of those bodies should be paramount, no?

In other words, if I am not actively paying attention to my body, then I am passively frustrating the Spirit's work, keeping myself from the renewal my mind so desperately needs.

Again, if you are an embodied soul, an embodied spirit—and you are—then you cannot tell where your body ends and your soul begins. No one can, including the most learned physicians and wisest philosophers. The fathers and mothers of the faith knew that only the Spirit of God can distinguish body from soul and soul from spirit. So, to put it sharply, even if you are relatively health conscious, you cannot be truly transformed without the self-awareness necessary to listen to your body and its wisdom.

Two Lifesaving Truths

I was running on empty for longer than I realized. I had been draining my internal spiritual and psychological reserves over the course of many miles crossed and many hours spent. When it all finally caught up to me, the timing couldn't have been more perfect, at least from the perspective of the enemy of my soul. The powers of darkness are always waiting for an "opportune time" (Luke 4:13). I knew how to recognize demonic activity, and I knew how to minister deliverance. I often taught on spiritual warfare. But my lack of self-awareness gave ample room for the enemy to overtake me.

Sadly, and with great regret, I came to discover the fragmentation, the gap, between my body and my soul. Now, on this side of my dark season, I have two statements that I return to again and again, statements I believe are lifesaving truths:

Slow down to the speed of life!
Slow down to the speed of revelation!

We tend to live in the fast lane. We want everything, and we want it now! If we must wait for it, it can't be worth it. We try to get everything done as quickly as possible. Because we've grown so accustomed to a life of instants, waiting has become foreign to us. We rarely "stop and smell the roses." Believe me, it is difficult to unlearn that urge to hurry and then slow down to the speed of life. And slowing down to the speed of revelation is equally demanding. Conditioned by the rapid pace of societal change and the exponential increase of knowledge, we live fast and furious, expecting and demanding everything immediately and in an instant. And we're mostly unconscious of how damaging that is to both our minds and our bodies.

Here's an example: My first computer was a Tandy from RadioShack. I remember the first time I tried to connect to the internet; I didn't know at the time how dial-up connecting worked. The first time I tried it, I heard all those strange noises for minutes on end, as it was seeking to connect, and I stood waiting until the connection was complete. Since the technology was new, my ten-minute wait didn't seem to be a big deal. At times the connection was lost, and I would have to start the process all over. But the reward of getting back on the World Wide Web made the wait worth it.

I was patient with how long it took for dial-up to work . . . *until* fiber-optic connections were perfected. Today, if it takes ten minutes to reach a website, I am beyond frustrated. Why? Because I have been conditioned to believe I can and should have that connection in an instant. My expectations and trust have been conditioned by my experience with this technology in all its rapid advances over the past few decades.

Contemporary Christianity is filled with clichés that are unfaithful and damaging to our bodies and our minds. I frequently hear professed prophets say they have received "a download from the Holy Spirit." In the early days of computer science and research, the term *downloading* found its way into the English language. It dates to 1975.[1] The term itself is defined as an "action or process of transferring from the storage of a larger system to that of a smaller one."

Notice, these are technical terms for mechanical objects. Because we live in a technocratic culture, we've borrowed these terms to describe human experience. This is tragic and at times borders on idolatry. As humans we are image bearers, not machines. We are embodied souls; therefore, the landscape of our interiority is spiritual, not mechanical. Metaphors drawn from that domain obscure the very nature of our being.

We Are Not Machines

Our psyche functions by the wisdom and complexity of the divine Artisan who shaped us to be breathed upon by the blessed Holy Spirit. Our cognitions, intuitions, imaginations, memories, reflections, and perceptions—all are influenced by our observations and have nothing to do with mechanics or technocracy. If we forget that, we lose the capacity to discern the impulses, the nudges, deep within the heart where God dwells. We lose touch with the movements of our own spirit where from the inside out the Holy Spirit influences our way of being, seeing, knowing, and perceiving. It is unfaithful, then, to say that God gives us "a download." It not only misconstrues our nature but also God's, reducing both God and us to storage systems.

Do you see how unholy this is? I am not a computer. I am not made of mechanical parts. My heavenly Father is not a massive storage system. So in order to be faithful, I need to know how to speak faithfully from a scriptural perspective about how the Spirit of God leads and guides us into all truth.

When I came out of my dark season, having had to deal with the dynamics of my entangled thinking, I began to learn not just how to slow down to the speed of life but also to the speed of revelation. What did that mean? It meant I had to learn to come to a place of inner stillness and watchful silence.

Over time, because I was ignoring the warning signals that my body gave me, I lost touch with my own heart. I gradually lost perspective and it became hard to remember *who* I was apart from *what* I did. So I had to learn all over again that it is only the watchful silence of contemplative prayer that brings me to a readiness to hear the deep, inner voice of my Creator—the Spirit of Christ, moving from the hidden depths of my inmost being into every fiber of my life.

I say all that as part of this detour because I know it was impossible for me to untie the knot of perplexity, apprehension, and anxiety until I owned that I felt that knot in the pit of my stomach and could not get rid of it! It was there morning, noon, and night—and all through the night. It contributed to my chronic insomnia and the need for medications, which didn't always work even though I took them regularly for a long time. Indeed, the medications are a story all by themselves.

You don't want to ask me about the "black box labels" and the possible negative side effects: I experienced them all! My anxiety and depression worsened. It was utter hell. But I found myself with no choice: I needed them as a bridge to heal so I could be "dialed-down" enough to find some relief and rest. My mind and body had to be reintroduced to each other in ways that were so foreign to my "normal" existence. Believe me, it was a *tough* pill to swallow.

My pride was devastated. I had to come to terms with the reality that my problem was not merely in my head but also in my body. I had to learn all over again how to present my body—and, if you will, how to be present *to* my body—as a living sacrifice, holy and acceptable to God. I had to learn to offer truly spiritual worship so I wouldn't be conformed to the elemental spirits of this world, and so I could experience the transformation of the mind that enables me to prove that which is good, acceptable, and perfect—the will of God! And trust me, beloved, that proving is a process, not a technique—a process of faith, obedience, and patience in suffering.

I am persuaded that most of us pay little to no attention to our fragmentation. We make excuses for it, presuming that grace glosses over it, ignoring the warnings of our own bodies, and running roughshod over many portions of the Sacred Text to justify our failure to be brutally and ruthlessly honest with ourselves and with God. We get locked in a vicious cycle, trapped on a treadmill of sorts, running fast but going nowhere; easily distracted, never maturing; never growing up, never showing up; quoting Bible verses as if we've arrived, all the while we're only amusing ourselves to death!

I began to realize in the middle of my dark season that I had to slow down to the speed of life and to the speed of revelation. I began to acknowledge the hard truths I had tried to ignore for so long. I began to break free of so many unhealthy and ungodly habits because I had been reminded by God's grace that

I live this life He has given me in a body that is imperfect and vulnerable, a body that needs to be taken care of and heeded.

Slowing down and paying attention made a world of difference. Thanks to my dream, which was a gift from the Spirit, I realized that the knot in the pit of my stomach would not go away until I was willing to accept its presence and to learn the deep, visceral realities it was endeavoring to show me. My prayer is that you will give yourself the space to slow down to the speed of life and revelation and listen. I promise, it will be worth it!

QUESTIONS TO PONDER

» How often have you ignored the signals in your body? What have been the consequences?

» What is happening at this season in your body?

» What are you doing about it?

» Apart from weekly worship in a local church (I pray that is part of your life and you haven't been so burned by the Church you have given up on it for a season), what are you doing for regular times of Sabbath?

7

The Knot in My Stomach

Sometimes all you can do is lie in bed and hope to fall asleep
before you fall apart.

William C. Hannan

In the quote above, William C. Hannan was reading my mail.
When I tell you I have been there, I am telling you the truth.
The chronic insomnia of my dark season, the constant fear that
the worst wasn't over yet, the knot in my stomach that felt as
if it would be eternally present and never let me go—all of it
plagued me incessantly.

Have you ever found yourself hopeless, saying things like . . .

"My head and my heart are currently a horrible place to
   be."
"I am so tired I feel like I need an extended break from
   life."

"I am so exhausted from having to be strong for everyone else, when I cannot even be strong enough for myself."

"I am just plain tired of everything."

When you're already hurting, you want to escape further pain at all costs. When Grandma or Mom ran hot water over my almost frostbitten hands and the circulation began to return to my frozen fingers, it hurt! In my dark season, I made matters worse by shaming myself for my struggles and for how I felt about the pain. I told myself, accusingly, that I should have known better than to let myself get entangled with my pain. So even as I tried to come to terms with the threefold knot in my stomach, I was tempted to utter the self-fulfilling prophecies of apprehension. My real issue, the real "thawing out" that needed to take place in me, was that my heart was deeply hurting, and the powers of darkness were present to do all they could to reinforce the lies.

Obviously, I am saying all this looking back. I didn't have this clarity and order in my thinking while I was going through hell. I had no idea where "normal" was, so I groped my way toward healing. All the while, I felt like I was out in the cold without the warmth and reassurance of the love I so desperately desired and the light I so desperately needed. I was so wrapped up in knowing what I thought I knew that I lost my sense of being who I was called to be, as a human.

What It Means to Be Spiritual

Beloved, being human is what it means to be spiritual. If you listen to too much popular teaching on spirituality, you get the sense that you are supposed to be angelic instead of human. But if God had wanted to make us angels, He would have. Instead, the divine Artisan made us to be and become fully and truly human. The Triune God said, "Let us make humankind in Our image and likeness" (see Genesis 1:26).

Christ became incarnate to teach us not how to be angels but how to be and become human. The most significant way in which He does that is by the way He taught us how to die, the offended One for all who offended Him. He died well because He loved well. He became, as the Nicene Creed says, "truly human." The implication is that because of the Fall, Adam and Eve lost their true humanity in the sense that they were estranged from themselves, at odds with the truth of their being, and so found they could not fulfill their calling. The powers of darkness dehumanized them. The knowledge they thought would make them like God in fact made them less human. It fragmented them and turned them into isolationists. The death and sin that entered their lives alienated them from God, themselves, each other, creation, and their calling.

We inherited that fragmentation. All the gaps in our lives that we experience inside and out are the result of what we inherited from our original parents. Oh, how much we need to be healed from the inside out!

I've been a pastor for a long time now. I haven't done it perfectly, of course, but it is my very life. I love the work of caring for others, nurturing them, and offering the support they need. God has graced me for that work. But being an empath means I'm highly attuned to the feelings and emotions of the people I serve, and that makes me especially vulnerable. Pastoral work requires rejoicing with those who rejoice and weeping with those who weep.

Yet in my dark season, when I could not find any rest, I entered into what psychologists call "hyper-empathy syndrome." Whenever others shared their pains, I felt coupled to their agony. Their suffering became mine—and not in a healthy way. I was so in tune with their emotional distress that I lived in a state of perpetual alarm, on high alert. The God-given boundary between self and other became somewhat porous, my sense of empathy lost its balance, and my well-being diminished quickly.

I couldn't disconnect from anyone else's pain, let alone my own. Worse, I couldn't tell where my pain ended and the pain of others began. It is one thing to put yourself in someone else's shoes. It is quite another to take their shoes from them for fear they won't be able to walk on their own.

Even though I was only forty-three credits away from my PhD in psychology, I could not diagnose myself. Afterward, however, I learned I was battling something called "personalization." That is a cognitive distortion, a type of negative thinking related to the way we assign blame for what goes wrong in our lives. Personalization is second nature for a dysfunctional New York Italian like me; my tribe wrote the book on dysfunction. I learned early on to blame myself entirely for every bad thing that happened, even when it was clearly not my fault. And when I did not feel guilty for things I hadn't done, I often believed that others did blame me. So often I felt I was the target of accusation and disrespect. Carry that kind of negative thinking over into ministry and it invariably leads to perplexity.

Beloved, we are human. All of us are fragmented and broken. We all wrestle with one cognitive distortion or another, even those of us who refuse to go to a therapist. According to the American Psychological Association's dictionary, a cognitive distortion is "faulty or inaccurate thinking, perception, or belief." And it occurs "in all people to a greater or lesser extent."[1] The dictionary provides "overgeneralization" as an example. An overgeneralization happens "when an individual views a single event as an invariable rule, so that, for example, failure at accomplishing one task will predict an endless pattern of defeat in all tasks."[2]

Losing Yourself the Wrong Way

Here is something we all need to realize: Although we routinely overgeneralize or personalize, in seasons of anxiety and despair we are much more vulnerable to such distortions, especially if we've suffered trauma. For me, the added weight of personalization was oppressive. It fed both the situational anxiety I was facing and the generalized anxiety I had developed over the months. Believe me when I tell you the powers of darkness used that added weight against me, trying to crush the last bit of life out of me. During my hellish years, the collapse of the San Jose mine in Chile happened. Late in the summer of 2010, thirty-three miners were trapped 2,300 feet underground. In the beginning, emergency workers had no way to communicate with them. Almost immediately, the government deployed a large rescue team, and the long, slow process of rescue began. The last of the miners wouldn't be saved from the mine until mid-October, however. It was touch and go for the entire length of the ordeal—sixty-nine days in all.

As you may remember, the story was all over the news, day after day after day. I had a very difficult time enduring it. The weight of oppression I felt was suffocating. Because of my hyper-empathy and personalization, it felt like every report I heard about the miners was happening to me. Oh yes, it was obsessive. I knew it was, which is why I didn't share what I was feeling with anyone. I was so frightened of what others might think about me. Still, what I experienced was unbelievably real to me, and indescribably painful.

I couldn't have known it at the time, but I was nearing the end of my awful season. The darkness that descended in July 2007 began to shift when the light dawned just prior to the 2010 Christmas season. By midway through 2011, I would be able to look back and say with Tramaine Hawkins, "My soul looks back in wonder how I got over!"[3]

I think of that time now as my own personal "three-and-a-half-year tribulation." Altogether, I was buried in that darkness for about 1,278 days, and I experienced little or no respite until the very tail end of the time. When the pain finally began to lift, it took another number of months to start feeling "normal" again—and the new "normal" was quite different from what I had known before. The good news is, as I adjusted to it, I found this new normal far more rewarding, meaningful, and fulfilling.

Certainly, some of our suffering is the result of our own folly and unfaithfulness. Yet not all of it is. In fact, much of it is not. Faithfulness doesn't always equate to prosperity, though the popular "feel-good" and "faith" messages try to convince us otherwise. How utterly untrue those messages are! Sometimes, as the book of Job reminds us, we "do everything right" and things still turn out "wrong." We need to be delivered from the magical thinking that keeps us from being and becoming truly, fully human. And that deliverance began for me in the acknowledgment of my pain and perplexity.

Paul, writing about his own dark season, tells us that he was "perplexed, but not despairing" (2 Corinthians 4:8 LEB). Trust me, I wanted to be there with him. But I wasn't. I was perplexed *and* despairing. He opens the letter by describing in some detail the spiritual and psychological impact of his suffering. He says he was "burdened beyond measure," beyond his limits, so that he actually "despaired even of life" (2 Corinthians 1:8 NKJV). Thus, later in the letter, when he says he is "perplexed, but not despairing," it seems clear, at least to me, that he has experienced some sort of release from the worst of the trouble. Somehow, amid his suffering, he gained insight into his perplexity and learned how to handle it.

With that hope in mind, let me talk plainly to you about my own experience. Let me disclose what I learned from owning that awful feeling in the pit of my stomach that I now "affectionately" (with my tongue in my cheek) call "the knot."

What's Too Painful to Remember

In the first chapter, I shared the story of our church move. The experience was intense and unnerving. I was stunned when our crosstown move prompted so many members to leave the congregation. As you might imagine, their departures came as a blow—not only to us as a church family but also to my sensibilities as a pastor.

I was so focused on what I knew—or what I thought I knew—about leading a congregation through difficulty, trying to convince myself that I was in fact capable as a pastor and a leader with some degree of influence, that my memories began to work against me instead of for me, demotivating and de-energizing me.

Really, there are only two kinds of memories: good ones and bad ones. I meditated on all the bad ones. This is what psychologists call *negativity bias*. And the more I rehearsed the bad ones, the worse ones I remembered. I knew that "what you focus on grows." But when everything looks and feels as though it is going horribly wrong, it is difficult to think about anything else! In that season, negativity bias became a survival skill and coping mechanism for me. My mind offered me a menu of bad memories from ministry experiences.

Truth be told, we're all far more impacted by negative events than we are by positive ones. Theologically speaking, that is because we live in a fallen world, which has left us fractured, fragmented, and in need of healing and restoration. We have been broken by suffering, pain, sorrow, and grief. Only the Triune God, who is love, can make us whole. Only God—Father, Son, and Spirit—can reintegrate us, healing the shattered and scattered aspects of our inner lives. Only the God who is love can reconcile us to ourselves and to one another the right way.

Even amid my perplexity, I believed God was good, all the time. I wrote a song back in the early nineties that went all around the world: "God Is Up to Something Good." It became a favorite in many "faith" circles. And now, in the middle of something that was decidedly not good, I had no idea what God was up to. It would have been easy for me to conclude that if

I'd had faith, this wouldn't have happened, or at least would've quickly turned out right. I knew that wasn't true. But I wasn't sure what was true, and with that perplexing reality pressing on me, my downward spiral began, my apprehension kicked in, and my anxiety began to rise.

That led to my becoming insecure about how people perceived me. I started worrying, almost obsessively, about being judged by others. Mind you, by this time in my journey I was known worldwide because of my television ministry. I'd had my share of detractors, and I'd learned how to shake off petty criticisms and keep moving. Now, however, criticism, whether real or imagined, struck like fiery darts aimed at my core (see Ephesians 6:16 NKJV). I started questioning myself in ways I'd never done. I wanted others to see me in a positive light, in a healthy light, in a "successful" light, if you will. I didn't want to be perceived as someone who, after all the years of bringing hope and help to others, was defeated by something he didn't see coming. Yet I had not seen the bus coming. It came, it saw, and it conquered—at least that's how it felt at the time.

Things were also changing in the contemporary Church at large. There was a movement away from solid and substantive teaching on Christ to the teaching of life skills and other self-help techniques. By that time, I already had more than ten thousand hours of certified and trained professional life coaching under my belt. I could have talked about leadership success, organizational achievement, and self-improvement all day long. Yet behind the sacred desk, I held a high value for the exposition of Scripture. I wanted to be faithful to tell the story of Jesus, rather than share cute stories in an attempt to make my ministry seem hip and cool. Still, I was troubled by the feeling that I was now in the minority of voices, and I felt as if I was no longer "relevant."

That word haunted me night and day during that dark season. How could I be perceived as having anything valid to say if I was not *relevant?* The nature of the contemporary Church sadly equates to "recency equals relevancy," meaning the more recent the insight, the more relevant it is. This is patently false and loaded with the wisdom from below, which the apostle James tells us is natural, earthly, unspiritual, and demonic (see James 3:15). At that moment, though, because I was perplexed, I became fused with those thoughts and began to see myself as irrelevant.

It seemed as though God had gone "radio silent." My apprehension kept growing the longer I was left in the quiet. While I would engage the Sacred Text, everything inside me felt formless and void, chaotic and unstable. The days of "let there be light" in my journey seemed long since gone, and I felt I was wandering in the perplexity of the dark void. That perplexity fed my apprehension, and the apprehension fed the anxiety—a truly vicious cycle.

Not all anxiety is bad. *Normal* anxiety is our body's response to stress. Any time you begin a new venture or are challenged to leave your comfort zone, you get anxious; that is normal. If you take an exam or if your boss notifies you of an upcoming job review, it's normal to feel anxious, even if you know you're prepared. As these examples show, normal anxiety is a *natural* sense of apprehension about something you know you must face. That kind of anxiety dissipates as you move through the experience.

But when anxiety causes you to live in a state of perpetual self-doubt and uncertainty, you know you're battling something *unnatural.* If you're constantly attacked by questions—"What if this goes wrong?" "What if that goes wrong?"—that's negatively affecting your health and well-being and is *pathological, abnormal* anxiety. The more it is present, the more intense it gets, and the longer it lingers, the more debilitating it becomes.

When full-blown perplexity became generalized in my way of thinking and feeling, the continual free-floating anxiety just about took me out. Traumatized, life lost all its joy for me. I felt detached from reality. I was merely going through the motions of existence, surviving, not thriving. In fact, I was only barely surviving. The pastoral pressures, the financial pressures, the paternal pressures, the sense of irrelevance, and all the other stressors showed up as one huge, confused knot in the pit of my stomach. It talked so loudly I could hear nothing else. But I still didn't listen to it. I had lost my way.

Learning how to listen to what the knot was telling me took a long time. But at some point, I realized I could only untie the knot by listening to it. The more I listened, the more I freed myself. Yet I have to tell you the truth: While I dealt with all these psychological dynamics, the powers of darkness were always there to hinder, harass, oppress, and annoy me. David said, "Even though I walk through the valley of the shadow of death, I fear no evil, for You are with me" (Psalm 23:4 NASB). I had to learn, as if for the first time, how God was with me in the valley of the shadow of death, where evil surrounded me. I had to find that banquet table where the body and blood of Christ could nurture and nourish me. I had to learn all over again how the administrations of the Word by the Spirit—God's rod and God's staff—were indeed my source of comfort.

The good news is that I am here to tell you the rest of the story, and to assure you that, despite any chaos you may be experiencing, God is with you. You will never cross the valley of the shadow of death alone.

QUESTIONS TO PONDER

» How attentive are you to the way your body responds to stress? How do you manage your body when you are moving through stress?

» How do you manage your body and your thoughts in order to relieve the stress?

» How often have you ignored the signals in your body? What have been the consequences?

» What is happening at this season in your body? What are you doing about it?

8

Going Out of My Mind

I have found that most people are more willing to accept physical pain and limitation rather than acknowledge and deal with the mental and/or emotional pain that might have caused it.

Tobe Hanson, *The Four Seasons Way of Life*

I want to be perfectly clear: While what I went through was only a season, it was a very long and painful one. Trust me when I tell you that it was no cakewalk. My victory was not easily won or won without cost. Quite the opposite. The strain, the pain, the seemingly endless struggle, the sheer exhaustion that came in my fiery ordeal was in many ways too difficult to put into words. At times, I honestly didn't know whether I was coming or going.

My mind was a battlefield. My thoughts, twisted like the knot in my stomach, were at war with each other and with me. I thought I had a pretty good handle on how the mind works, but what I had to walk through challenged all my previous deeply

111

held assumptions. I don't say this to discourage or dishearten you. I say this for one sole purpose: You may be in the exact same place and feel as if you have no hope. You always have hope, because God is the God of the impossible, the God who makes a way when there seems to be no way.

I lost my appetite for a long time. The knot was eating away at me. I dropped twenty pounds. Not only did I not want to eat, but the very thought of food intensified my pain. This left me in a "catch-22." If I didn't eat, I couldn't replenish my already-weakened physical state. I had to learn to force myself to eat. This was certainly not me. I'm a foodie, a New York Italian whose middle name could have been anything from Pasta to Cannoli. Now, everything lost its appeal. Life itself had lost its taste for me.

But that proved to be only the tip of the iceberg. My mind was being torn in opposite directions. Due to the agony in my stomach and the torment in my head, my body remained in that perpetual state of fight-or-flight that I've already mentioned. Given the nature of the knot in my gut, the very physical indication of the extreme anxiety that plagued me, my mind was endlessly barraged by fears, including the obvious concerns for my health. How could I go on living if this intense emotional and psychological pain did not subside?

The Many Faces of Anxiety

If you could find my high school yearbook, you would see that my classmates and I each had some kind of motto under our pictures. Mine was "Rule your mind or it will rule you!" I was all of seventeen years old when I claimed this as my life motto. I had no idea how little control I had over what would happen to my body and what would come into my mind. When trouble found me, it was as if the fountains of the deep in my unconscious opened and the floodgates burst into violent torrents of confusing thoughts. Though I tried to operate in a constant "damage control" mode, I couldn't keep up with the damage. My body never relaxed. My mind never rested. The turmoil was present and relentless.

In addition to free-floating anxiety, I also experienced situational anxiety because of the many troubling circumstances that converged in that season. There was no place for me to turn and find any peace. Truly, none! Situations that normally would never have stressed me out now seemed like mountains of oppression looming large over my consciousness, mountains that refused to be removed.

Under normal circumstances I would have been able to differentiate between what was happening and who I was as a person. But my mind had become so overwhelmed that I didn't know where I ended and the pain began. It felt as if I had no mental defenses left. I am not sure I can fully describe that kind of experiential state in words; I can only say that the psychological pain was excruciating. Yet . . . I still had to function. I still had to travel to make a living. I still had to preach and lead a congregation. I still had to sustain a television broadcast that was aired literally worldwide, and I still had to show up for my family.

Traveling became extremely difficult. Sitting still in a small space for hours on end, my already-beleaguered mind running away with itself, was no mean feat. It took all the concentration in the world just to sit at the table for a meal or ride in the car to church. Mind you, I had been on the road and sleeping in hotel beds for years. So I knew how to adjust to sleeping less and sleeping less well. Now I was robbed of sleep almost altogether.

At home, I at least had the comfort of being in my own bed and the relief of feeling no pressure to awaken at a given time and no pressure to act in any performative way once I was awake. On the road, however, I had to perform, and at a high level.

All of this meant I dreaded more and more having to be on the road. Acutely aware that everyone around me was going about their lives in a normal fashion, anxiety and negative thoughts constantly badgered me. The heaviness of carrying that weight left me feeling totally helpless. I worried that at any given moment I might just collapse in front of everyone and fall apart.

You won't be surprised to hear that trying to maintain the appearance of "normal" took everything I had to give and more. I was running on fumes. Imagine then having to prepare and deliver sermons. Each week, I dreaded the constraint and tension that arose as the weekend drew close, knowing I had to prepare sermons and deliver them to the congregation on Sunday morning. I couldn't run. I couldn't hide. Week after week, month after month, and year after year, I had to stand in front of the congregation, feeding them from the Scriptures, and assuring them that God's faithfulness was their portion, all the while feeling as if these were empty words coming from a desolate soul. I had grown mostly numb living in survival mode. But when I stood behind the pulpit to preach, I felt a spark; I was somewhat clear. When I was not in the pulpit, however, the dread, the angst, the terror, and the darkness would return with immediacy and ferocity.

All that notwithstanding, I knew I had to stay in touch with what was most valuable, most central. I had to learn how to function somehow when it would have been preferable to "curse God and die" (see Job 2:9). When I was home, I would sit for hours in the dark, or lie on top of the bed as still as possible, hoping perhaps that sleep would return, even during the day. I tried to wrestle with the notion of what it meant to walk "in hope against hope."

I wanted to hear from God, but it was difficult. "Be still, and know that I am God" (Psalm 46:10 NKJV) was an impossibility during that season. The stillness evaded my grasp. I had known it in my past. I had known the pregnant silence of the presence of the living God. Yet in the darkness that descended in the middle of my life, the experience of stillness was nothing but a distant memory, far removed from the reality I was enduring. I feared I would never find that place of stillness again, and that fear only made me sink deeper into despair. Even the promise of living "in hope against hope" became more than anything a taunt.

The Friend Who Sticks Closer Than a Brother

I did have one companion who was constant and competent: Vinnie. We'd been fast friends since our days in Bible school, and by the time I was going through this season, we had known each other more than thirty years. I do not know what I would have done without him and the way he interacted with me in my pain.

Vinnie knew how to help me cope. He became my travel partner, sitting up with me through endless nights. When we were not on the road, he was available by phone morning, noon, and night. He helped me navigate my way both at home and away, in the public spotlight and my private hell. His compassion and care provided a path toward promise and hope, even when that path seemed to be blocked by many obstacles and fraught with many unexpected threats.

While seeing a therapist was helpful, it was Vinnie's pastoral brilliance, his understanding of Scripture, his personal walk with God, and his unconditional love for me as a friend that proved to be my best help in time of need. When the agony first began, Vinnie got on a plane and stayed in the house with us, to be present and available to help me make it through. His sense of humor saved me in the most maddening moments, breaking the tension when the torments of hell were so intense that I felt I wanted to die.

Vinnie helped me remember who I was, reminding me how to smile and laugh. He listened patiently to my complaints—at a time when I felt even God wasn't listening. Unlike Job's friends (who were fine as long as Job remained silent), Vinnie could handle my pain when I spoke about it. He had the patience of a saint. If I asked a question once I'm sure I asked it a thousand times, but he never tired of repeating himself. And as far as I can recall, his answers were always fresh and lifegiving, empowering me ever so slowly—and I do mean *slowly*—to regain my perspective.

If I had the power to confer a doctoral degree in clinical psychology and pastoral theology in relation to the human condition and how to manage it well, I would confer it on Vinnie. He wasn't afraid of my pain or of how I talked about it and processed it. He gave me permission to be ruthlessly and brutally honest. Mind you, he was my favorite teacher in Bible school in part because of his stories of faith and miracles. He knew God could move in ways that bring healing and deliverance; this was a matter of fact for him, not speculation. He served a God of signs and wonders. Yet he was also ready and able to climb down in the trenches with those who were suffering, to listen fearlessly to their pain.

Vinnie also knew how to use the ministrations of the Scriptures, the "rod and staff" of Holy Writ, to comfort the afflicted. He did that for me throughout my entire years-long journey in the darkness, present with me every step of the way. I had learned a lot from him long before I went through that season, but as he walked with me in the worst of my sorrows, I benefited even more from him.

Vinnie's words, always fitly spoken, drew out of my silence the layers of pain that were robbing me of my well-being. And he didn't only speak to me, he also spoke *with* me and *for* me. As each layer of fear was unearthed and exposed to the light, he prayed me through to God, again and again.

I cannot say enough good about my friend. But I can say this: Vinnie's presence was for me the healing presence of Christ.

When I couldn't hear God, I could hear Vinnie—and he sounded a whole lot like the God I had known. If you asked me then, "What does God's voice sound like?" I would have said, "Vinnie." For all I had learned, all I had preached, all I had taught, and all I had prophesied, I still desperately needed a friend who would stick closer than a brother.

Vinnie was that and more. He acted with the wisdom of the Great Shepherd. He led me to the streams of living water where God restored my soul. Whatever else is said about him when he stands before the judgment of God, Vinnie will be honored as a good shepherd and faithful friend to me.

Vinnie certainly wasn't like Job's friends! In the next chapter I explore the story of Job. His self-disclosure of his pain, as revealed in his speeches and recorded in the Sacred Text, proved to be a vital help to me in my journey. My internal experience seemed so eerily like his. And as you would expect, when you're in hell, every opportunity to find a clearing and room to breathe is like coming upon an oasis in the dry and barren desert.

Job's friends did not answer his complaint righteously, but Vinnie enabled me to be as open, as transparent, as honest as I needed to be. He gave me permission to find my voice in my pain. Job's friends looked to expose some secret sin they were convinced Job refused to own. But Vinnie looked for *me*, trying to help me find where I had gotten lost in all the hell I was going through. Job's friends were better off when they sat in silence for seven days.

Today, I have a sense of what Job suffered, a feeling about what was going on in his heart and mind amid his dark season. But I also have something Job did not: the story of a friend who did not speak faithlessly or accusingly, but graciously walked me through the worst of my suffering and pain.

Beloved, when it feels as though you are going out of your mind, you will be tempted to isolate. I understand the temptation. It is not easy to invite people into your chaos, because it means that others will see you at "your worst." Please realize that such experiences are part of the human condition and not a cause for shame. Such shame is not godly but demonic. When you are suffering, God can use the right friend or friends to come alongside you. Allow Him to work through them. It is part of His design—the Body of Christ.

QUESTIONS TO PONDER

» What person, whether living or deceased, has loved you no matter what? How did their love help you?

» With whom are you able to be totally transparent and not be looked at in a demeaning way?

» If you are in pain right now, what conversations might you need to have, and with whom? If you aren't having those conversations, what steps are you prepared to take so that you will have them?

9

A Dark Night of the Spirit

In the dark, thoughts become louder.

Mie Hansson

Job sat in the ashes—the ashes of the daily sacrifices he offered for his family to the living God, the Creator, the God of Abraham, Isaac, and Jacob. In Job's days of well-being, those ashes served as a sign of his faithfulness to God, his long trust in the righteousness and justice of God, his steadfast care and concern for his entire family. Now, after the calamity, those same ashes gathered beneath his pain-racked body offered no solace. In fact, they mocked him. They became burned-over memories, the remains of a former life, a better day.

Where Job had once been and where he now found himself were impossibly far apart, and the difference was too much for his mind to reconcile. He went to reach for a memory, a memory of his loved ones, his ten children and their families, and all he could find were the cold ashes left by what he sacrificed for them.

For Job, these were the ashes of death itself. His pain seemed to him utterly unbearable. His wounds seemed utterly incurable.

How do you process such pain, grief, loss, and agony? How does anyone bear to sit in the ashes of sacrifices made for loved ones now gone, sacrifices now known to have been wasted? How could anyone live with knowing that they themselves are actively being reduced to ashes, ground into the dust from which they were made?

Job's appearance was so changed by his agony that his friends didn't recognize him. When they showed up, they saw something that would find ultimate fulfillment in a Man who was beaten beyond recognition on a cross outside the walls of Jerusalem: "Just as there were many who were astonished at him—so marred was his appearance, beyond human semblance, and his form beyond that of mortals" (Isaiah 52:14). Job's friends didn't recognize him. Worse, he didn't recognize himself. And I can tell you firsthand, although perhaps you already know it: When the pain is so great and the suffering so intense that you can't seem to recognize yourself, you've descended into what the psalmist calls the pit, the deepest depths of the darkest darkness.

I hadn't lost a loved one, let alone ten children. But I did face deep, deep pain within the life of one of my sons, pain that, of course, affected our entire family profoundly. And as I've shared with you already, that pain, added on top of all the other sorrows that had fallen on us at the time just about took me out. A mountain of challenges weighed on me, body and soul. I felt I was being crushed, slowly suffocating from the mounting pressures.

I would not claim to know exactly what it felt like for Job to sit in the ash heap. I do know, however, that I felt everything I had worked for, everything that mattered to me, was being consumed by a fiery ordeal. I know that it felt like I was suddenly living a present that made my past seem like another person's life altogether. I know I didn't recognize who I had been, and I was frightened by who I felt I had become.

When I first began to wrestle with the agony, I could not say, as Job did, "The LORD gives, and the LORD takes away. Blessed be the name of the LORD" (Job 1:21 csb). Oh, I taught and preached on that passage many times. I said things like, "The surest sign that God is going to give you something new is that He takes away what was formerly given that has outlived its purpose." That line was a crowd pleaser. It was sure to speak to those who were going through hell and high water, sure to give them a boost to trust God's work in them and on their behalf. Sadly, that line is only half true, and I was totally insensitive to what was really going on in that "the Lord takes away" moment in Job's life.

It's easy to preach about Job when you haven't suffered what he suffered or sat with him in the ash heap. Consider all he lost. Consider all he endured. Consider all he had to undergo. Then, and only then, consider his amazing confession of God's goodness and justice despite it all. Job lived from the inside out in a place where I could only hope to live. Scripture says that he didn't sin with his lips (see Job 1:22). I cannot say that about myself.

The events of September 11, 2001, changed history. We know that's true because we think of time as being divided by that day's events. We talk about the world as it was before 9/11 and the world as it is after. In the same way, my dark season was the time that divided my life, marking out a clear "before" and "after." I remember lots of things about life before my dark season. Yet lots of things seem vague because my sense of self-awareness has changed so radically. I thought I knew who I was prior to my dark season. I suppose I did know to some degree. But I never once expected that by the time I hit fifty, the "midpoint" of my life, I would have to face a total disorientation, a violent disruption of all I had known as "normal." Now I can see more clearly. What began in the summer of 2007, just prior to my fifty-third birthday, would dramatically alter the trajectory of my life, setting a new course for me and my ministry.

During that long, protracted season, I had to maintain my normal schedule. One night, I was hosting a live roundtable discussion on TBN with various prophetic voices. Having to chair the dialogue took all my strength. Sitting in one place for more than a few seconds usually proved impossible, because the nervous tension coursing through my body forced me to keep moving. The powers of concentration necessary to maintain some semblance of poise, appear "fine," and carry on a meaningful conversation sapped whatever was left of my depleted resources. The guests had no clue; the audience in the studio had no clue; the audience at home around the world had no clue, but I was not well. Nonetheless, even there, even under those circumstances, God was at work, making things known to me.

That night John Paul Jackson was sitting immediately to my left. He has passed on now, but at the time I counted him a friend. Many knew John far better than I did, yet we had interacted at several national events and built a relationship that was precious to me. I had wanted John on the show that night because of his insights into life in the Spirit and the way he himself had learned to walk through difficulties.

During that season, John talked about a perfect storm he had just come through. At one point he turned to me, not knowing what I was enduring, and said something to this effect: "Mark, we both know what it is to endure a dark night of the soul. However, we also have had to endure a dark night of the spirit."

Clouds and Thick Darkness Surround Him

Theologically, the phrase "dark night of the soul" carries significant weight. It originated with a sixteenth-century Roman

Catholic mystic, Saint John of the Cross. Saint John wrote a lengthy poem under that title to describe the soul's journey from its beginnings in our human, broken condition to its home in God. For him, the dark night of the soul was tied to the difficulties, tests, trials, and hardships the psyche endured in being weaned from the world and brought closer in union to the God who dwells in unapproachable light.

For the mystics of the Church, knowing God is understood in terms of what cannot be known, what cannot be formulated in words or formed in concepts. Paradoxically, mysteriously, the God who knows us, the God who makes Himself known and knowable, cannot be known. He is hidden even in His revelation. This is called apophatic theology, and it requires us to think and to speak with deep humility. God, these mystics teach us, is to be approached from a place of not-knowing. This is what the psalmist called us to understand when he cried out, "Clouds and thick darkness surround Him" (Psalm 97:2 NASB), and this is why the prophet reminded us that God's thoughts and ways are unlike ours: "As the heavens are higher than the earth, so are my ways higher than your ways and my thoughts than your thoughts" (Isaiah 55:9). And this is also why the apostle reassured us of the hope we have in Christ: "Eye hath not seen, nor ear heard, neither have entered into the heart of man, the things which God hath prepared for them that love him" (1 Corinthians 2:9 KJV). For Saint John of the Cross, the closer we get to God, the more mysterious our knowing of Him becomes.

This way of knowing in and through *not-knowing* is necessary in part because our senses have been compromised by the Fall. Not only our physical senses—the way by which we process what we see, hear, taste, touch, and smell—but also our spiritual senses. Our spiritual eyes and ears and nose, as well as our feel and our taste must be purified so that we can know God truly. We must be weaned away from the natural light that has governed the way we believe the world works so we can become acclimated to the Uncreated Light who is God Himself.

Thus, according to Saint John of the Cross, the closer we get to the God who cannot be known, the darker our experience must be. The light cannot be truly seen until we've entered fully into that dark, embracing it as the nearness of God. That, basically, is what is meant by "the dark night of the soul."

Before we get back to what John Paul Jackson said to me in our roundtable conversation about the "dark night of the spirit," we also must consider the complement to apophatic theology, which is cataphatic theology. Generally, this way of thinking appeals more to the Western Christian mind because it begins with what can be known about God and uses positive terms to describe Him. It is rooted in the confidence that what God is believed to be can be thought and spoken. So, for example, to say that God is love from a cataphatic perspective is to make a confession we believe we can trust as true. If apophatic theology urges us toward awed silence, cataphatic theology urges us toward songs and shouts of praise.

Both ways of doing theology are necessary. Both are essential to what I learned in my dark season, drastically changing my outlook and altering the trajectory of my life. Each is strengthened by the other. By His very nature, God is unlimited and beyond knowing.

When we study Scripture and Church history, one of the first things we learn is that as much as we think we know about God, there is so much more we don't know. In popular contemporary Christian experience, however, we're liable to lose touch with the not-knowing, the silence that makes our knowing and our speaking trustworthy. We want our theology not only to be clear but to be quick and easy. We like having an explanation for everything that happens. We like believing that we have a handle on how God works. That has a lot to do with our need to be in control and very little to do with the nature of the mystery of the Triune God. We like it because it gives us a false sense of being able to overcome uncertainty.

Sometimes, we actually behave as if God lives in the box we've constructed from our ideas about Him. We try like mad to hold on to our ideas and opinions about how God works, but many of them have nothing whatsoever to do with Him or with how Scripture reveals Him. That is somewhat understandable, given the major convulsions the culture is going through and the many shakings that are taking place globally. But we need to ask ourselves, "What if God Himself is the one shaking everything that can be shaken?" Know this: God cannot be put in the box, and God will break whatever boxes we make for Him.

We don't get to choose whether we want to embrace an apophatic approach or a cataphatic approach to God. It isn't either/or, it's both/and. Orthodoxy means "right believing," and orthodoxy is full of paradox. That's why the Scriptures are filled with all sorts of contradictions that can't be reconciled, at least not at the surface level. Those apparent contradictions are there on purpose because God knows we need them. The Spirit put them in the Scriptures to teach us how to come to terms with who this God is whom we worship. They are God's way of accommodating our human weaknesses, frailties, and the limitations of our finite minds.

For example, when the Scripture says that God regretted making human beings (see Genesis 6:6), we must ask ourselves in what sense that is true. How is it possible that a God who knows the end from the beginning wrestles with regret? Nothing takes God by surprise, and God is not at the mercy of emotions the way we are. God always knows everything perfectly without having to think about it. That is what it means to say that God is omniscient, or all-knowing. This text, then, forces a puzzle on us because it makes a claim about God that seems wildly inappropriate and unfitting.

125

The ancient teachers of the faith knew that when the text speaks in such strange ways, it is because there is a deeper meaning or hidden sense that we need to seek out. The Scriptures are designed to bring us to the place where we must search out an understanding of this mysterious God who hides so we will seek Him.

First Samuel 15:11 tells us that God regretted making Saul king. Yet earlier in the book we're told clearly that Saul was God's choice. All this gets confusing, doesn't it? And since we're going to talk about Job, let's wrestle with this difficulty, too: the Scripture is very plain when it says that "all have sinned and fall short of the glory of God" (Romans 3:23 NKJV). Solomon says almost the same thing in Ecclesiastes 7:20: "There is not a righteous person on earth who always does good and does not ever sin" (NASB). But remember that the book of Job opens with this claim: Job was "blameless and upright" (see Job 1:1).

How is it, if all have indeed sinned, that Job is blameless and upright? To make matters worse, God later confirms the judgment, telling Satan that Job is indeed blameless. But that raises another question: Why is God allowing Satan to appear in the courts of heaven in the first place?

Why a "Dark Night"?

Before we look at Job's story in more depth, we need to return to what John Paul Jackson said to me out of the blue, live on the set, about the "dark night of the spirit." I was still enduring it, of course. But his statement intrigued me, even in my pain. Apparently, even amid my anguish, a part of me could still interact, function, reason, and wrestle with the truth. I wasn't completely dead inside or numb to the Spirit. Despite everything—the chronic sleeplessness, the knot in my gut, the free-floating anxiety, the crushing despair—I retained a portion of my interior life and continued to seek and wrestle with the paradoxes confronting me. Though my wrestling looked different, I still attempted to "make sense" and "make meaning" of the madness that was my portion in that season. In the darkest depths, the Spirit kept my spirit alive, if only barely.

In the days that followed, I decided to search out the meaning of that phrase, *the dark night of the spirit*. I found it was linked to Job's story, and that those who used the term linked it directly to a familiar passage in Hebrews 4:12–13:

> Indeed, the word of God is living and active, sharper than any two-edged sword, piercing until it divides soul from spirit, joints from marrow; it is able to judge the thoughts and intentions of the heart. And before him no creature is hidden, but all are naked and laid bare to the eyes of the one to whom we must render an account.

Hebrews is a book of "betters." It teaches us that the New Covenant is better because our High Priest and Mediator is better, and the Mediator's blood speaks a better word than the blood of bulls and goats. We know from other New Testament passages that Christ is Himself the better Word (see John 1:1; Revelation 19:13), sent from the Father to accomplish our redemption and the redemption of the whole world (see 1 John 4:14). "The Word of God" is not something He became but is His title, which denotes what He has always been. He is the Word who speaks, and the better word that comes from His mouth is like a sharp two-edged sword (see Revelation 1:16). Thus, we can see that the Word He both is and speaks is living and active, because He is the I Am that I Am—the living God! Isaiah says that when God's word goes forth from His mouth, it never returns void (see Isaiah 55:10–11). So when Hebrews speaks of the two-edged sword, it is a reference to Christ as the Word who speaks a word that *does* what He *is*. What He says to us and about us and over us is deeply penetrating, dividing what is seen from what is hidden in the secret recesses of our being.

All of that is glorious, but we should not be glib; the two-edged word of God cuts clean and deep—that is exactly what radical surgery requires. And in the early stages of my painful season, God performed radical surgery deep within my interiority. It took me a long time to realize what was happening. And even as I learned to trust through the pain, I never came to enjoy the process. At times I wished the Lord would take me home. Who wants to undergo deep surgery while awake?

It was anything but a convenient time for my life to be interrupted. I had too much going on that I needed to attend to. Things were falling apart around me, and I had to be at my best to navigate my way through it. The all-penetrating gaze of the all-seeing God exposed everything to scrutiny, and He didn't ask permission. The two-edged function of His Word operated like a surgeon's scalpel on the heart of my heart. At times I recoiled, because I wanted to think there was nothing left in me to be exposed. I was past all of that . . . wasn't I? I detested the notion of "weakness, in fear, and in much trembling" (1 Corinthians 2:3 NKJV). But God did not let my frustrations stay His hands.

When we look at that portion in Hebrews that speaks about the dividing of the soul and the spirit, we can find it easy to think the author is speaking of two separate realities. That isn't quite the case, however. Notice I said, "not quite the case." There is a *distinction* between soul and spirit, but no separation. You've heard the saying, "I am a spirit, have a soul, and live in a body." But that is not true to the meaning of Scripture. Our way of reading, which lacks input from the original languages and the context in which those words were first used, makes the Sacred Text seem to say something that it is not saying.

Some ideas, like that popular saying about spirit, soul, and body, get passed around in our circles as unquestioned truths.

In our circles, the moment someone claims, "The Spirit told me thus and so," who dares question them? They are claiming divine authority. And they are speaking to people who are predisposed to think that those who claim to speak with authority are telling the whole truth and nothing but the truth.

People speak as if they have the authority of the Spirit, even when their way of approaching the Sacred Text is mistaken. Often, they're ignorant of the original languages, and they rarely bother to go back and discover how the early doctors of the Church maintained the ways in which Jesus taught the apostles to interpret Scripture.

The problem is, when the only measure of truth is how "spiritual" we sound, we can make the text say anything we want. We've been conditioned to think that if we go into our prayer closet, read the Scripture, and notice some detail in the text that we find remarkable and exciting, we have had a "revelation." John, Peter, Paul, and all the rest of the apostles would shudder at that kind of thinking. They knew better.

We should know how Jesus taught His disciples and how they then taught their disciples so that faithful ways of reading the Scriptures were faithfully maintained generation to generation in the churches. That kind of work no longer seems important to many of us, unfortunately. We're too caught up with being "relevant."

Hebrews does teach a distinction between soul and spirit, to be sure. But if it doesn't mean the kind of separation assumed by the popular teaching "I am a spirit, I have a soul, and I live in a body," then what does it mean? Can we know what it means without knowing how those terms were used in the Church's history and in the ancient world?

The Greek word for soul is *psuché*, and the Greek word for spirit is *pnuema*. These words were used in the ancient world as synonyms. Josephus (who died AD 100) and Philo of Alexandria (who died AD 50), for example, asserted that the terms are virtually identical. Is there a legitimate reason to think this is true in our Scriptures?

There is. According to the Septuagint, the Greek version of the Old Testament, God breathed *pneuma*, which is breath or spirit, into Adam, and he therefore became a *psyche*, a living soul. The late G. E. Ladd, a much-loved professor at Fuller Theological Seminary and someone deeply familiar with the ancient languages and the history of Bible translation, explained that "recent scholarship has recognized that such terms as body, soul, and spirit are not different separable faculties of man but different ways of seeing the whole person."[1]

What we call the "mind" today also has a different connotation than it did in the ancient world. It had to do not with the head or the brain but with the heart. Remember, Jesus says that our thoughts come from our heart, not our head. We tend to think of mind as where rational thought takes place, but for the ancients it was the seat of personhood and selfhood. In fact, many scholars argue that the Hebrew *nephesh* and Greek *psyche* are better translated in those terms. In the New Testament, therefore, the term *psyche* implies an overall sense of who a person is.

I take time with this example to show why it's important to understand what these concepts meant when they were written so we don't impose on them a contemporary meaning that obscures the intent of the Sacred Text. So "penetrating the division of soul and spirit" isn't about the setting apart of two separate things but about the setting side by side of two ways of describing our integral interior lives, ways that God alone by His Word can expose and lay bare as distinct.[2] "Joints and marrow" refers to the exterior, physical, and material parts of our being. Ultimately, then, the writer says that the purpose of Christ and His Word are to expose and scrutinize the thoughts and the intentions of our hearts, laying bare the truth of our selfhood, our personhood. The real issue then is this: None of us can escape divine scrutiny. God sees who we are and knows all there is to know about us. In more common vernacular, when it comes to God, we can run but we can't hide.

What I think John Paul Jackson wanted to share with me in that moment was that God was doing radical surgery in me, scrutinizing the deep places hidden from my view, places that needed to be brought into the light. I think he recognized this because he had endured a similar season and had undergone a similar scrutiny. He too felt like Job and sensed somehow that I was now in my own time of trouble.

Later John Paul told me that during his dark season he just sat and stared out the window for hours on end. He said he didn't have much to say and found it difficult to understand what was transpiring. His personality was different from mine, so for him the issue of anxiety might not have been as intense or as pronounced. Still, the similarity between our experiences was uncanny.

When he shared this word for me, however, I knew I wasn't about to go looking for what was wrong with me. That was surely going to be a dead end and far from a healthy posture. But I also knew I had to learn to deal with what was there in the depths, triggering the unrest. And I could do that work because God was doing something deep and trustworthy. When I see John Paul on the other side of the eternal divide, I will embrace him and thank him for his love.

Dark nights of the spirit don't come and go without getting our attention. At the very least, they compel us to look in and look up. If we are willing to do both, the God who is spirit will expose our depths and heal them.

QUESTIONS TO PONDER

» Are there some areas of profound pain—either emotionally, psychologically, or physically (or all three)—that you are facing currently? If so, how are you talking to yourself about them?

» Again, as before, get in touch with your self-talk, and write down what you are telling yourself about all of this. As you read what you have written, what do you notice on paper that is different from what you assume in your mind?

» In which of these areas might the truth be less present than it needs to be?

» How would you reframe those thoughts in a way that exposes them to the truth?

10

I Won't Complain. Or Will I?

Wisdom comes alone through suffering.

Aeschylus

Beloved, suffering is real, and all of us suffer to one degree or another. In the struggle, it can be difficult to keep a clear head. Our emotions get stirred, our circumstances become unsettled, and we feel pressed from every direction. Some of our thoughts are raw and unrefined, coming straight from the depths of our pain. We can either stuff those thoughts and serve our misplaced notions of faith, or we can face them honestly. That means owning them and taking them to God, who knows our thoughts before we think them. He is touched with the feeling of our infirmities and is big enough to handle our pleadings and—yes—our complaints. How else can we be healed? Can we run to Him and leave our brokenness outside His gates?

I propose that we cannot. A vital part of the Job narrative is the man's transparency before God. Job articulated his hurt, confusion, disappointment, and anguish—his honest, human complaints—before God, much as David did in the psalms. God responded and restored Job, but not because Job's faith was bulletproof or free of all doubt. It was because Job came as he was and stood before God as *He* is. Job's approach was not methodological but relational.

Job accepted his emotions and voiced his concerns to God, based on what he knew about Him and His trustworthiness. You might say that Job was guileless and openhearted toward his Maker. He was therefore receptive to God's ways and willing to lay himself bare before Him. This posture left him open— not to Band-Aids and quick fixes, but to the deep providential healing that works from the inside out.

With that in mind, I based this chapter not on methods but on the biblical and theological realities that sustain the lives of those who believe. These realities are not microwavable or reducible to three, five, or seven steps. They are real nourishment, forming us and our responses to God and moving us toward the healing we all crave.

Allow yourself to chew on these truths. You will have questions, and you can ask them. God can handle them! He desires to be known and allows you the space you need to reach new places of understanding along the way. Wrestle with what you are about to read. Let it reveal things about God and about you—things that might not have occurred to you before. As you do, I believe Job's story will speak to your own and help you to articulate your concerns—your complaints—to the One whose love redeems.

Know Your Adversary

Job's transparency stands in stark contrast to the duplicitous nature of another figure in Job's story. He is called "the Satan,"[1] a sinister adversary whom Jesus named as a liar and a murderer from the beginning. There is no truth in him at all, nothing in him that is reliable, except that he always shows up to hinder, harass, annoy, and destroy. Out of his own awareness that his time is short and the lake of fire awaits him, his goal is to bring into his own destruction as many of God's creatures as he can. "Misery loves company," as the adage says.

If we look at the figure of Satan from a psychological perspective, we recognize that he sees everything through the lens of his own corruption. So when he accuses both God and Job, he is only projecting his own corruption onto them, as if they are guilty of what he himself is filled with.

The book of Job contains many riddles to solve. The story itself is a large poetic parable and riddle. The justice Job's three friends speak of and seek to live by is known as "retributive justice." They're convinced that it's the divinely sanctioned order of the universe. Their wisdom resonates with portions of the Torah and Israel's wisdom literature, to be sure. But remember, orthodoxy contains many paradoxes. While there may be texts in which retributive justice is spoken of, many other texts do not tie justice to retribution at all.

So the real question about what's going on in the book of Job is how a good God can allow evil to touch the righteous. It's a tough question and not an easy one to answer. I've heard countless sermons by preachers who have Job all figured out. Most of those who claim this aren't Hebrew scholars and have no idea of the ways in which most English translations fall short of the Hebrew. Yet we buy into their conclusions without wrestling with the text for ourselves. To put it bluntly, we tend to go to church to get our needs met rather than to know God. We prefer our ears to be tickled rather than to be told the truth that leads to sanctification.

But without pastors proclaiming the truth, we remain enslaved to the adversary's lies. At times, our minds are minefields filled with cognitive distortions, generalizations, willful gaps in knowledge, and areas of blind deletions resulting from our refusal to see what we need to see. That our brokenness is so pervasive shows that we need time with God, something beyond a moment at an altar or five minutes of morning devotions. The healing presence of Christ, the healing Word of Christ, is an ongoing "Let it be." And that word takes the whole of our lives (and beyond) to fully appreciate. Even on the other side of the grave, when we get home to glory, He will have to deal with our unfinished business and "wipe away all tears from [our] eyes" (Revelation 21:4 KJV).

Heaven is a place of great rejoicing, but the promise that God will wipe away our tears implies that when we get there, whatever we didn't cry through, groan through, or agonize over in this life will be brought to the surface in the presence of the One who is the truth. He is health and life, and He searches the heart and tests the mind. There, He will address the disintegration left from our brokenness.

Before we will ever be able to enjoy heaven for the gift it is, we will have to lay down all our burdens by the riverside, as the old gospel song says. So if John the Revelator is telling the truth, we will have to cry just a little bit more when we get to glory. And then we can laugh.

Works in Process

Beloved, all of us—and I do mean all of us—desperately need healing. All of us are fragmented. All of us are broken. All of us have been diminished by what took place in the beginning in the Garden of Paradise. All of us need deliverance. All of us need to be loved. All of us need salvation. And we need it constantly, day to day and minute to minute.

Salvation isn't accomplished in a moment, but over the course of a lifetime. Salvation is a Person, just as the truth is.

His name is Jesus, which means "Jehovah is salvation." And if we are going to read Job from the perspective of this Jesus—and He said that all of Scripture is talking about Him—then we need to ask, "Where is Jesus when Job is in the ash heap?"

The writer of the book of Job crafted a marvelous work that reveals a hidden wisdom, which must be discovered through the process of a searching interpretation. The writer tells us that a conversation occurred in the courts of heaven, without Job's awareness. I'm pretty sure it would have helped Job to know that his name came up in the throne room, and it would have helped for him to know that an out-of-control bus was careening toward him. But that never happens for any of us—not only because our enemy never tells us the truth and not only because we can't hear the Holy Spirit perfectly, but because it's rarely if ever good for us to know what's coming.

Of course, there are times the Spirit seeks to alert us. But our ability to discern what the Spirit is saying is flawed. Remember the many times both before and after the resurrection that the disciples thought they had it all figured out—and missed Jesus altogether. "Oh," some folks say, "We've got all that sorted out now. We have the fullness of the Spirit and perfect revelation. Everything we see and hear from the Spirit is crystal clear. We have a direct pipeline to the mind of God. All we have to do with doubt is rebuke it."

Some folks really do think that way. They believe they aren't susceptible to the errors of the many disciples who doubted at the resurrection, doubted at the ascension, and made mistakes after Pentecost. They think they are much more advanced than the apostles and saints of old. If that's the way you think, throw yourself a party. But be careful: What the adversary will be celebrating is how thoroughly he has deceived you. He will toast your delusional thinking and your misunderstanding of Scripture and the tradition of the faith. I say that not to shame you or anyone who falls for his tricks. I say it to remind us of our fragmentation and to evoke a renewed awareness of our need for deliverance and healing.

Most of all, I say it so we don't forget the good news: God is ever patiently at work to heal us, taking all the necessary time to free us from the primal fears that wreck our lives. Jesus, by the Spirit and on the Father's behalf, continually works in us to strip away every mask of shame and false pretense. He is delivering us from the fear of rejection and invisibility, and He labors to bring us face-to-face with His glorious Father, in whom there is no shadow of turning.

The Sacrifice of Sorrow

Job didn't get a preview of coming attractions. You could say he was doing everything right, yet suddenly everything went horribly wrong. He didn't see the bus coming. Oh yes, he was concerned for his family. He was concerned that they might curse God. He knew the nature of our human condition. He knew his own brokenness, and he knew the brokenness of his loved ones.

Job was a descendant of Esau. The text says he was a man "of the East" (Job 1:3 NKJV)—not an Israelite and not a descendant of Jacob. The East was the inheritance of Esau and his descendants (see Genesis 10:30; Job 1:3). Yet even as an outsider to the covenant, Job knew the truth about what it means to be human. And he lived well—better than anyone else, in fact. But that did not save him from the season of darkness. Trouble found him, as it finds all of us, eventually.

Remember, Jacob received the blessing, not Esau. Job, as a man of the East, wasn't a son of Abraham and didn't share in the covenant God made with Israel. Yet this son of Esau believed in Abraham's God, loved that God, and was loved by that God. He faithfully offered sacrifices to that God because he had an innate sense of God's justice, righteousness, holiness, mercy, love, faithfulness, and goodness. Job was faithful to the God who was known for His faithfulness.

And God knew Job! Do you remember the Lord's own testimony of Job, spoken to the devil himself? "There is no one like him on the earth, a blameless and upright man who fears God and turns away from evil" (Job 1:8). What an astounding claim: "There is no one like him on the earth"! Don't you want to ask in response: "God, are You forgetting all the patriarchs who were in covenant with You prior to Job's arrival?" Don't you want to protest, "God, are You forgetting the faithful saints in Israel who were in covenant with You at that time?"

Why did Job stand out? What was it that God found so remarkable in him?[2]

The Hebrew Scriptures began as an oral tradition, which was passed from generation to generation before being written down and gathered into a collection. When it was all sorted through and assembled in three parts (Torah, the Prophets, and the Writings), the exiles were in Babylon, awaiting their release at the end of the captivity.

The story of Job serves a special purpose in Israel's story and bears particular significance for the exiles in Babylon who, unlike many of their fellow countrymen, chose to live by the water. When the rest became absorbed in the Babylonian culture, these exiles continued as a righteous remnant sitting by the river and weeping over the memory of Zion.

But why did they sit and weep?

They were plunged in an extremely dark season. They had thought their holy city, the home of their hope, would abide forever. Yet it burned to the ground and lay in ruins.[3] Everything they worked and lived for—everything they had built—was gone in a moment. Left without their temple, priests, and sacrifices, they saw little to do but hang their harps on the weeping willows beside the rivers of Babylon and weep for all that was lost.

So that is what they did: They sat and wept without a song.

You must remember what weeping was for the sons of Israel. But you also mustn't forget the meaning of the river. Psalm 119 is a teaching psalm designed to instruct the worshiper of Yahweh in the wisdom of Yahweh. It includes this declaration, an intention of devout service: "Seven times a day I praise you for your righteous ordinances" (119:164). Another psalm instructs worshipers to wash their hands, literally and figuratively, each time they pray: "I wash my hands in innocence, and go around your altar, O LORD" (26:6). According to the Law, the priests in the Temple could not offer sacrifices or lift their hands to pray unless their hands had first been ritually washed and cleansed. This habit was handed down as an ordinance from God to Aaron and his sons, and all Hebrews were taught to take it on as a necessary practice.

So why was the remnant in Babylon weeping at the river? How does it relate to the story of Job sitting in the ash heap after the death of his children and the loss of his fortune? How does all of that relate to me in my dark season? How does any of it relate to you and the trials of your life?

There was a time when the prophet Joel admonished the priests to "weep between the porch and the altar" (2:17 NASB). This instruction came after a series of plagues from locusts that had eaten up all of Israel's harvest. When the locusts descended and devoured the crops down to the roots, God essentially offered to take His people's weeping as prayer. According to the word of the prophet, they had only to put themselves in the right place and give vent to their sorrows. Though they had no words left, they did have tears. So they offered them as prayers, as living sacrifices.

In my own dark season, as I told you, the knot in my stomach was eating me up. Like the plague of locusts that ate up Israel's harvest, something was devouring me, and I couldn't get it out of my gut. But I eventually learned to do what they did: I had to throw myself down between the porch and the altar, weeping and uttering my honest complaints before God. There was no perceptible turning point—no light that suddenly turned on or "revelation" that kicked in. It was a process of change within myself that was unique to my inner life and personality. You could say that understanding gradually dawned on me and moved me toward the healing I desired, even as my pain persisted. I learned something of the deep truth in that old song "Tears Are a Language God Understands." He understands the words spoken from our pain, too, assuming we can find words in our suffering.

The exiles in Babylon wanted to be faithful but no longer had a temple and no longer could offer sacrifice; they found themselves exiled not only from their land but also from the glory, the Shekinah, that had dwelt over the Mercy Seat between the wings of the cherubim in the Holy of Holies. So they gave themselves to cries and tears. All they had left was the voice of their sorrow—their lamentations, their mourning, and their griefs. But because weeping in lamentation is a legitimate form of prayer, and because prayer requires clean hands and a pure heart, they chose to live by the water. They wanted to pray without ceasing; that meant living in the only place where they could wash their hands in running water continually.

The Lord had given, and the Lord had taken away. But the right of the covenant assured them that if they found no words but could only offer their pain through cries and tears, they would be heard and remembered by the God who had shown Himself faithful to their ancestors. Their moans and groanings were more than enough to make a sacrifice. Amid their agony, they knew that they needed to remember the God of Israel who hears the cries of His oppressed and makes a way out of no way. That God had a history with their people, so they sacrificed their tears to Him.

The book of Job mattered so much for them because his story fit with that long history of God's faithfulness. Though it was written generations before the exile, probably by a stranger to the commonwealth of Israel, Job's suffering, pain, agony, and intercession spoke to the hidden depths of the insiders' experience in exile. It opened them up to a justice that was too good to be retributive and served as a peculiar witness to the only hope exiles have: the hope that seems against all hope.

Not All Complaining Is Bad Complaining

One of my favorite songs, "I Won't Complain," written by the late Rev. Don Johnson, still touches a deep place in my soul. Many great artists have sung it over the years, including Marvin Sapp, Karen Clark Sheard, Donnie McClurkin, Clay Evans, and Paul Jones.[4] But I especially loved the way Bishop William Charles Abney Jr. performed it.[5] Bishop Abney pastored Bethel Pentecostal Church in Grand Rapids, Michigan, and we became good friends. Not long before his departure from this life, he visited our congregation in Orlando. I didn't realize he was there until I got to the pulpit. Recognizing him, I asked if he would be willing to sing "I Won't Complain" for us.

By that time, Bishop was on dialysis, yet he was entirely gracious and affirming. He came to the pulpit, and I went to the keyboard and started in his key. Needless to say, he wrecked the house. The words he sang are available online.[6] They talk about trusting God through life's ups and downs, even in moments of doubt or confusion about the way forward. In writing them, Reverend Johnson recognized God's faithfulness and promised not to complain about the tough times.

During my dark season I was so flattened emotionally that I rarely wept. Not that I didn't want to cry; I simply couldn't. Even my groans were stifled. I had lost my cry. I simply ached until I was numb, which left me absolutely perplexed and seemingly incapable of voicing my anguish. But Bishop's singing of that song always reduced me to tears. Why? Because it articulates both the doubts and the trust hidden in the secret places of my heart, hidden most of all from me.

That said, something in those lyrics needs to be questioned. It is not the part about trusting in the Lord and boasting in His faithfulness. It is the part about *not complaining* to God. When your troubles seem too heavy to bear, voicing your complaint to him is neither wrong nor bad. The psalms teach us to do that very thing, and so does Job.

In that hardest stretch of my life, a line from the opening chapter of Job caused me great trouble. Honestly, it left me intensely afraid, and now I know it was because of a poor interpretation: "In all this Job did not sin or charge God with wrongdoing" (Job 1:22). The Satan could not trap Job into cursing God. Job knew that to curse God would be to "sin with his lips."

At times, of course, our sins do get us into trouble and cause a great deal of suffering for others. But it is a mistake to think that whenever we experience trouble or undergo suffering, we must trace its cause back to some wrongdoing. To think that way is to do what Job's legalistic friends did. Driven by a need for retributive justice, they pried into his life, perhaps imagining that they cared for him. But it seems clear that they were seeking for reasons to justify what befell him. They were seeking confirmation of their views, not the comfort of their friend.

While we point out the failures of Job's friends, we need to be cautious and remember that, in the end, they acknowledged their wrong and repented of it. At any time, any one of us can fall into the trap of refined legalism. Many of our churches encourage it. Some who boast the loudest about walking by faith in fact walk by sight. And because they see the world legalistically rather than spiritually, they use the letter of Scripture to kill and maim themselves and those around them.

The same is true of the magical thinking that has left so many people hurting, lost, and languishing in our churches. They've finally discovered the formulas don't work. They've discovered God isn't their errand boy. All they have left are questions: "What did I do wrong?" "Why didn't God answer my prayers?"

I am not afraid of these questions or scandalized by such doubts. I am not disgusted or disappointed with those who find themselves at a loss. After what I endured, I no longer look at the Body of Christ in the same way. I see "lost sheep" as truly distressed and downcast, harassed and helpless, desperately in need of the Great Shepherd, exactly as I was. And I hope to do whatever I can in His strength to feed them and tend them so they can come to know His healing presence. But I know that a great many people are disgusted and disappointed with anyone and everyone who struggles or complains. I'm afraid our churches and our communities are filled with Eliphazes and Bildads and Zophars.

We need to remember that faith always works only by grace, not by technique or procedure. Faith is not some secret knowledge. That is a gnostic idea by which the "favored few" hope to assure themselves of better outcomes and happier lives.

Sadly, I know many Christians who think that way. They're a lot like Job's friends. Of course, they never think of themselves in those terms, but they treat the suffering people around them as though their pain is, by definition, their fault. They assume that trouble comes and stays only for those who either lack the "revelation knowledge" that guarantees healing or the "holy boldness" to force God to do what they want.

Those who teach these distortions are often celebrated. Instead, they need to be confronted, and their teachings need to be condemned. Such thinking does unspeakable damage to the hearts and lives of the saints and the reputation of the Church. We need to take stock of ourselves! How easily we fall prey to perverting the truth and embracing deception from the powers of darkness. How easily we damn the saints who are suffering most when what they need from us is patience and encouragement.

As I shared earlier, I had a true friend in Vinnie. He gave me permission to bring my complaint to speech, even when I was afraid that my complaining would be sin against God. But trust me, Job's friends also showed up during my dark season. Some seemed delighted to see me in pain because they felt I deserved it. Others felt I needed to be humbled. Many distanced themselves because they didn't want to be identified with anyone who claimed to walk in faith but wrestled with profound pain.

It's a tough lesson to learn, but not everyone has your best interests at heart. In your very worst moments, when you're walking through hell, you find out who your true friends are. You also find out about the false friends, the ones who claim to be blessed and highly favored and then reject anything that challenges their opinions—notice, I said "their opinions"— about how God works.

In the end, God sharply reproved Job's friends for their hubris, false teaching, and judgmentalism (see Job 42:7–9). They intended to correct Job and "adjust" his theology, thinking they were justified in doing so. They tried to convince him that he did not know God or himself. But God expressed His wrath against their lies, in no uncertain terms: He declared that they spoke unfaithfully, but Job spoke rightly. God even required them to seek Job's intercession and forgiveness.

It's not that God left Job's thoughts entirely unchallenged, but He seems undisturbed by Job's complaints to Him. Is it faithful to promise, "I won't complain," as the song title suggests? Remember, the lyrics were written after a long season of reflecting on life's tests and trials. They came after the storm was over, and God's goodness was on full display. I'm sure that if we could speak beyond the grave to the late Bishop Abney and ask him whether a complaint ever crossed his lips during his weary days and sleepless nights, that great man of God wouldn't hesitate to admit the truth. I can almost hear his response: "Son, do you think I wasn't human?"

We want Jesus to be like Superman—a God who isn't vulnerable, who doesn't bleed. We want God to be like that because we want to be like that ourselves: untouchable and invulnerable. But Jesus doesn't fit the bill. If we look to Christ crucified, we see that He has entered fully into Job's experience. Golgotha is His ash heap. So look at Him bleeding on that cross, crying out the words of Psalm 22:1, "My God, my God, why have you forsaken me?" Then ask yourself: Was He sinning with his lips?

Of course not! No, this was God Himself weeping "between the porch and the altar." This was God Himself offering a lament. This was God complaining. And in it all, God was teaching us to weep, to lament, and to complain. This is God doing for us exactly what true friends always do, especially in the darkest times: He was giving us all the time and space we need to heal.

QUESTIONS TO PONDER

» How well do you verbalize your sadness? your anger? Describe the difference between describing your feelings and venting them.

» What might the relationship be between the ability to live in the present moment without distraction and the ability to verbalize your pain well?

» What do you think happens to you when you choose not to bring your pain to speech? What might happen if you began to write down your pain so you can describe it better?

» What are you prepared to do so you can begin to move forward and not allow your pain to get in the way of what matters most?

11

Power and Powerlessness

I am living in hell from one day to the next. But there is nothing I can do to escape. I don't know where I would go if I did. I feel utterly powerless, and that feeling is my prison. I entered of my own free will, I locked the door, and I threw away the key.

Haruki Murakami, *1Q84*

Implicit in Job's story and every account of human suffering is the reality of power differentials—the real or perceived inequities in how power is distributed between and among the story's characters. In any given life situation, we either feel empowered or powerless. How we feel can be anchored in reality or colored by what we learned about power differentials during our formative years. Based on those lessons, we can feel empowered even when we are underdogs. Or we can feel utterly powerless when others think we have it all together.

Part of Job's struggle was tied to the sense of powerlessness he experienced during his trial. Meanwhile, in his quest to discredit Job, the adversary wielded whatever power was available to him. When the Lord praised Job, the adversary denigrated Job's character. Because the Lord had confidence in His servant, He permitted the adversary to test Job's loyalty.

Thus, God afforded the Satan some power to conduct his test by inflicting pain and suffering. When Job passed the first test and refused to sin with his mouth, the Satan received a second opportunity to afflict him. We tend to oversimplify what happened in the opening scene because we want to avoid the difficulties it presents. There are mysteries in this text. Job's friends were sure they knew the reasons for Job's sorrows. But he avowed his innocence and insisted that his suffering could not be punishment for wrongdoing because he had done no wrong. The more he claimed innocence, the more they declared his guilt and urged him to acknowledge his sins.

Why? I propose that they were convinced of how the world works. They believed in the predictable pattern that "everything happens for a reason" and "the punishment always fits the crime." While passages in Scripture speak of this aspect of justice,[1] Job posed a challenge to these assumptions. And in the end, God declared that Job was right and his friends were wrong.

The Satan suspected that Job served the Lord for personal gain. He raised the cynical question: "Does Job fear God for nothing?" (Job 1:9). I have been in pastoral ministry now for many years, and I have known some who served God for personal gain. While that is not always the case, it is a reality for some who profess Christ. Yet this certainly was not the case with Job. The adversary contended that if Job's many blessings were taken away, Job would curse God to His face.

The question at the core of Job's great trial is this: Does Job serve God based on the favors he has received from God or for the sake of God alone? This question and its answer are why the Lord allowed the trial to take place at all. Scripture tells us that Job was a remarkably pious man whom the Lord valued highly. The Lord knew his heart inside and out. So in raising such a cynical question, the accuser impugned both Job and God. If Job served God for selfish reasons, then he wasn't truly serving God at all. And if God was unaware of Job's infidelity, then God Himself was a fraud.

British evangelist Mike Darwood, a precious friend from the beginning of my faith journey, once explained in a service that God allowed this trial. Darwood believed that Job was God's man on display before an accuser—and the trial would prove the accuser false. Job knew that loving God meant loving Him for who He is, not for what He gives. He knew that serving God out of that kind of love meant no reward would be expected or needed in return. He did, in fact, love God for Himself. Even on the ash heap, having been stripped of all that he considered dear, Job offered worship and blessing to God. And in the process, he exposed the contempt of the accuser and the errors of his accusing friends.

My dark season dramatically changed my perspective on this story. More than ever, I cherished Job's willingness and boldness in making his complaint known to God. That honesty in prayer became essential for my own mental health and well-being, just as it had been for Job. As I have learned from the extensive work of Old Testament scholar Walter Brueggemann and the great Eugene Peterson, faithful prayer brings *everything* to speech, not only those things that seem pious and acceptable to the religious.

Job's so-called friends recoiled at his insistence on his innocence because for them everything happened according to the dictates of justice. No one suffered unjustly. No one was rewarded without reason. Nothing absurd or meaningless ever happened. *Many* Christians believe the same, even now. And that is why they act exactly as Job's friends did. They are, as I said in the previous chapter, refined legalists, experts in the letter that kills and ignorant of the Spirit who gives life. They have learned to read the Sacred Text with natural eyes, void of the Spirit's inspiration.

151

Remember, Saul of Tarsus knew the Scriptures well before his encounter with Jesus, and he used the Scriptures to justify his animosity toward followers of the Way. He also hated Jesus, inflicting suffering on Jesus' followers in the name of Yahweh—all based on his interpretation of the Sacred Text! That is a warning: We can make Scripture say anything we want, and until Christ Himself opens our eyes, freeing us from those falsehoods that corrupt our readings, we will never interpret it faithfully.

One thing to keep in mind as you read the story of Job: The Lord is large and in charge. When the Satan appeared in the court of heaven, the Lord was seated and enthroned as Sovereign King and addressed the accuser from a place of absolute authority: "Where have you come from?" (Job 1:7; 2:2). During the second interrogation, the text mentions nothing from the accuser's lips about what had already afflicted Job. Instead, the Lord brought it up. Why? Because what already unfolded proved the adversary wrong. Still, he refused to own his delusional thinking in the presence of the Sovereign God.

This denial of the truth led to the next event of the trial. The accuser hated the truth because there is no truth in him. And the Lord wouldn't allow that kind of deception to stand in the court of heaven. So He brought the accuser face-to-face with his flawed thinking and slanderous character, and He did so by acclaiming Job. Job was still the Lord's servant, still blameless and upright! Because God knew Job's character, He allowed the Satan to fail dramatically, exposing once and for all his vanity and the futility of his attacks.

How the Truth Prevails

My somber season enforced upon me a fresh appreciation for how the truth prevails: It triumphs no matter what it faces and no matter what opposes it—but it takes time. In a world of "instants," where we want everything right now—microwaving or DoorDashing our meals and Googling our questions for immediate answers—abiding through difficult, painful processes proves trying. When James invited us to consider the "endurance [patience] of Job" (James 5:11), he sought to make us aware that transformation often, if not always, happens slowly and even agonizingly. The goodness that God works into the depths of our being takes time, and time can only be experienced moment by moment. Depending on how deep the work is, abiding patiently is essential. We must not be enslaved to the clock or driven by the desire for quick fixes and immediate turnarounds.

My three-and-a-half-year ordeal was dull and drab, gloomy and overcast. Excruciatingly aware of the ticking clock, I was desperate for the season to end. The powers of darkness offered me false interpretations of reality, which were tempting because God seemed silent and absent. If God was "pleased" with me during that season, I couldn't feel it. Yet God was working things out at a level deep below my conscious awareness.

It is difficult to assess whether Job had much of an understanding about how the powers of darkness were arrayed against him. We know he felt he would not survive, and that God was against him. I didn't think I would make it, either. And I surely didn't think I was being perfected by grace or that God was going to vindicate me, proving I was safe in His arms—not just safe from the accuser but also from my own pained and broken heart. When all hell was breaking loose, Vinnie often—and I mean often—quoted this verse to me: "The eternal God is your refuge, and underneath are the everlasting arms. He will drive out your enemies before you, saying, 'Destroy them!'" (Deuteronomy 33:27 NIV).

I'd forgotten about this teaching that Job was God's man on display, which I'd heard in the early years of my journey with Jesus. But in the darkest season of my life, the Spirit brought the conversations between God and the accuser to mind again and again, leading me to this idea that I, too, was God's man on display. Still, it was difficult for me to believe that was true. If I was God's man on display, I sure didn't feel like it. I felt like a miserable, totally flawed, failure of a human being.

We can glean a lot by paying careful attention to the story of Job, particularly in relation to the ways the invisible realities (including the presence of evil) interact with and impact our daily lives. I had to deal with all the ways in which the powers of darkness assaulted my well-being. I had to contend with the "flaming arrows" (Ephesians 6:16) of the evil one. I realized that my own thinking needed to be reevaluated, because the enemy was using my interpretations of my experience against me. Yet the ultimate objective of the lesson we learn from Job is not what the Satan is allowed to do but rather who God Himself is and what God will ultimately reveal in us and accomplish through us.

I tended to take mental shortcuts regarding the demonic prior to that ghastly season. I assumed that I knew enough about the Scriptures, God, the accuser, and evil spirits. I thought I had everything figured out, sorted neatly into tidy little boxes of understanding. I thought I knew enough to maintain control of what was happening to me. I was wrong, and I had to learn how wrong I was. This presumption was tied to my avoidance strategies and defense mechanisms. I also felt overmatched by what was happening, so I grasped for whatever power I felt I had, trying to use it to navigate my way.

Disempowering Presence

In the book of Job, the accuser possessed a certain amount of power, which the Lord affirmed (see Job 1:12), things given into his "hand" (Job 2:6 NKJV). We cannot forget that. We wrestle mightily with issues of power. Growing up in a dysfunctional world, from the time we are children we learn that we are powerless in relation to those who are over us and stronger than us. For others to be bigger than us, to tower over us, is more than a physical reality. Our perceptual filters are affected at the deepest levels by these experiences of weakness and vulnerability.

I was no different. Growing up, what I learned about "power" was that I didn't have any. I loved my dad dearly, yet that does not change the fact that my relation to my father shaped my sense of powerlessness. In that sunless season, I had to face my deeply held assumptions about power, and I had to own my sense of powerlessness, all of which stemmed from my relationship with a man who had himself always wrestled with feeling disempowered.

At the midpoint of my life, I reached my limit. Like Job, I found myself sitting in my own ash heap. Like Dante, I found myself in a dark wood at the mouth of hell. I honestly felt as though the powers of darkness had swallowed me up. I had been riding high. You could say I was successful, but "success" is such a fleeting, arbitrary notion. Who decides what it is? Who determines whether you've achieved it? Does being crucified on a dung heap outside the walls of Jerusalem, cursed as someone lower than the beasts, spat upon, and mocked as He cried out in agony, "My God, My God, why?" constitute success? Or to ask the same question another way, what kind of power was Jesus displaying when He was crucified in weakness?

That season in the dark wood threatened me with the loss of everything I felt I had accomplished. I had "arrived," yet not without struggle. My achievements had been "hard won." But what did I actually "win"? What now was I so afraid of losing? I was at the mercy of what I thought I needed, yet it was also taking my life, little by little. I was deeply torn. If I wasn't relevant any longer, all I had accomplished by the time I was fifty seemed a waste. If, as I feared, the rest of life was a downhill trek, why had I worked so hard for so long? What had been the purpose for moving on? Had it accomplished anything other than wearing me down to nothing?

Let me take you into my history a bit more deeply. As I already said, I was an only child, and I was expected to live up to my Italian father's heavy expectations. His own dreams had been shattered—or more to the point, foregone—so he wanted to relive his life through mine. He had to forego his dreams for the sake of his father's dream. Dad wanted to be a doctor. He had been two years into a pre-med program when he was drafted during World War II and had to put his education on hold.

Grandpa built a coal and ice business during the Great Depression. Back then, the furnaces in homes were coal furnaces. Refrigerators weren't on the market yet, so people had "iceboxes" that looked like fridges but had a compartment at the top for a large box of ice, which kept everything in the lower cabinet cool. By the time the war was over, coal furnaces became oil or gas furnaces, iceboxes became refrigerators, and air-conditioning units became available for homes. Grandpa had developed quite a few customers who were ready for in-home heating and cooling systems.

So when Dad returned from the Battle of the Bulge, Grandpa told him he had to take over the family business, because he was the eldest son. Dad needed to go back to school—but not medical school. He was to enter business training so he could oversee the full transformation of Grandpa's coal-and-ice business into a home-heating fuel and air-conditioning business.

Let me take even a further step back now, to another important detail in how my life unfolded. As the oldest of seven brothers, my dad had a brother who died at just under two years of age, and Dad felt responsible for this death. This was his deepest wound, and he carried the scar his entire life, though he never talked about it and became angry and shut down emotionally if anyone ever mentioned it.

Dad and his younger brother Mike were tasked with watching their baby brother, Vito. One day, while Grandma ran around the corner to buy groceries, they were babysitting him. Dad was about twelve at the time, and Uncle Mike was about ten. A huge pot of water filled with lye had been left on the stove to boil because Grandma intended to scrub the floors when she returned. Vito managed to escape Dad's notice for one quick second and tipped the pot of boiling water over, scalding himself to death and scarring my father's psyche and conscience for life.

When I was a child, Dad rarely if ever let me out of his sight. He was always preoccupied with my health; every sneeze and sniffle caused him to rush me to the doctor. Though I didn't understand it at the time, he suffered a sense of guilt and shame that marred every aspect of his life. Fear had gripped his mind. To make matters worse, he also had major issues with his own father, who expected him to take care of the family because he was the firstborn son.

Dad also saw the strain on his mother, who had to raise seven sons. When he was still a boy, Dad protested on her behalf. My grandfather, the stereotypical Italian patriarch, slapped him in the face for daring to question him. Dad, who had his own father-wound, vowed that when he got married, and if he had children, he would have only one child. He hoped that child would be a son, and I was that son.

I can see clearly now that whatever the power differentials were in the family system, Dad felt powerless even while he was forced to carry out the responsibilities of the eldest son. I can also see how and why my father's father-wound drove him to act in ways that wounded me and left me feeling powerless. He had lived with his brothers, but I had no siblings to share the pain with, which made the power differential in our house even starker. Dad had all the power in our relationship, and because of his own brokenness, he clung to it tightly.

Any attempt I made to grasp for power was met with a forceful rebuke. When I questioned whether I wanted to be a medical doctor, for example, his answer was as quick as it was sharp: "You will be a doctor." I had no choice, no personal power. Since he'd had to give up his dream for Grandpa, he surely was not going to let go of it now that his son could fulfill it.

From the time I was old enough to be aware of myself, this feeling of powerlessness, born of the knowledge that I had no choice about my future, instilled in me an entire series of reactive patterns, which I would not come to terms with fully until the middle of my life.

On this side of that midpoint, I see that whether or not we care to admit it, we organize our lives around fear, especially the fear of death. Over the years, as I reflected on my memories, I recognized how I had organized my life this way. Yet it took me a long time to learn that I had accepted my father's fears as my own. My ego boundaries weren't strong enough to dissociate his fears from mine, so his became mine. Without knowing it, without asking for it, I inherited my dad's brokenness. And I didn't know how to dissociate who I was in that regard from who he was. Dad carried himself as if he were fearless. But every time he was angry, that anger was a mask for his fears. Unconsciously, I absorbed that hidden fear whenever his anger showed.

We might not like to admit it, but we all have a certain degree of compulsory behavior. And I have learned that wherever compulsion and reactive patterns are present, fear is the driving force. I know I had developed from early childhood several avoidance strategies and defense mechanisms, albeit unconsciously. And I adopted them for a reason: I felt I needed to protect myself because I was at the mercy of my father's power.

Now I know better what I was feeling then and why: I had been stripped of my sense of personal power. Personal power refers to the ability to have the decisive say in our own lives, the capacity to be influential and to make a difference.

Is there something in your heart that dreams of making a difference in the lives you touch? That is born out of your confidence in your personal power, and it begins to present itself when you're quite young. I would argue it is the direct result of God's work in your life.

Of course, the older you get, the more responsibility you have to take on. At first, I had to learn to study, keep up with my chores, and manage my allowance. Later, I had to hold down a job—in the family business, believe it or not—while excelling in school. I assumed various roles and responsibilities during the summers of my high school years, helping my family as they serviced furnaces and air conditioners and delivered home-heating fuel to their regular customers. I had to learn how to answer "up" to my uncles. I was a novice; they were the experts. Though I was not entirely powerless, the power they exercised was far greater. Later still, I took on other jobs, working as a short-order cook, a waiter, a busboy, and a piano teacher. In every one of those roles, I had to answer "up" to others. In each role, I discovered basic power differentials.

In any relationship or set of relationships, there is a power differential. And much depends on how power is managed and negotiated. I learned again and again that no matter how responsible I was, no matter how faithful I showed myself to be, I was never good enough to earn any power from my father. Therefore, I developed a profound distrust of the little personal power I did have. Not only that, I also developed a deep suspicion of others, which affected all of my relationships. I began to think that anyone in my life who had more power than I did would use that power to remind me of my powerlessness. I was deep into my thirties before I determined that I didn't want to live that way any longer. And that is why I keep saying that what we fail to deal with in adolescence we will be forced to deal with in middlescence.

My dad and I had our first "come to Jesus" encounters in my late thirties. I did indeed rebel against my father's authority when I was a teenager, but my rebellion got me nowhere. By the time I was a grown man, however, I realized I needed to let Dad know the pain I carried, even though I knew it would be challenging. It was painful for him to hear. He denied my pain, and my memories of the pain, in every conceivable way. We argued a lot, especially in the beginning, and the healing took *lots* of time. Yet even after the relationship was healed, and irrespective of my accomplishments, acquired skills, and wisdom, the deeply embedded image of my overbearing father continued to haunt my dreams. Ironically, that image has always shown up in the visage of my actual father, though I had to learn through the dark season that it was an image I had taken as my own. I had confused that archetypal image of my father with who I was and how I was to be.

It took years for me to realize that the archetypal dream-image of my father and my real-life dad were two different realities. For so long I could not distinguish one from the other. Because of the ways I had been formed from my youth, I had ingested that image and taken it to myself as an appropriate image for relating to and dealing with myself.

As I've mentioned, one of the factors that pushed me into my dark season had to do with one of my sons. Even though I knew, intellectually, that what was happening was not a result of anything I'd done or left undone, I felt like a failure. My sense of fatherhood was called into question, which is not surprising, given the way I was raised. When you're used to being blamed for everything that goes wrong, including things that are entirely outside your control, it is easy to develop the habit of indiscriminately blaming yourself. I had said for years prior to that fateful season that circumstances don't make us or break us, they only reveal us. And yet it wasn't until that bus finally ran me over that I unearthed all kinds of hidden pains.

Those early lessons I learned about others' power and my own powerlessness profoundly impacted my cognitions, perceptions, emotions, feelings, reactions—and yes, the knot in my gut. I had to reckon with how small I felt on the inside when I was called to look like I was standing tall on the outside. So many times, I felt smaller than I really was and felt I needed protection when I wasn't in any real danger. I had to face all those insecurities to stare down the fear of power and powerlessness that had controlled so much of my life.

Where Are You When I Need You?

The bus ran me over four years after my father died. During the dark season that followed, I missed him terribly. I longed for him. I desperately wanted to know if he'd ever experienced such pain. Had he felt this kind of anxiety? Had he fallen into despair? Since he was the more powerful of the two of us, he always seemed to be "in control." I yearned for his presence because I felt he might know how to guide me through the darkness, or at least offer me the light of his own testimony.

But it was too late . . . he was gone. Despite our reconciliation, my lack of familiarity with his internal struggles left a deficit in my soul as deep as the Grand Canyon. I wanted so badly for him to tell me how he had processed his fears as a father and how he had felt during those stressful situations I saw him face as the head of the family business.

I was able at times to read the pain on my dad's face, yet he never disclosed the pain in his heart. He was part of a generation that didn't talk about such things. As a man raised in a patriarchal culture, he had learned to "suck it up" and keep going. Looking back, knowing what I know theologically and psychologically, I would contend that he had repressed a lot.

He had buried his most painful memories, and with them his most troubling fears. The challenge is, when you bury that stuff, it's still alive and kicking, and at some point, it comes back to bite you.

It indeed came back to bite my dad—right around his fiftieth year when he lost everything, including the family business, and began to self-medicate with alcohol. Mom endured great pains in that season, and I grew even angrier with my father because of how he was handling himself. I know now that he was a bundle of distress. Yet in the midst of my own hard time, when I most desperately needed whatever wisdom he had learned from his trials, he was not there. His secrets died with him. And the fact that he had survived his own dark season, seemingly without any dependence on or help from God, only deepened my sense of powerlessness.

Though he was gone, the image of the disappointed, tyrannical father stayed with me. It loomed large in the deep recesses of my psyche, swelling as my darkness grew darker. Mind you, I knew we had reconciled. We had affirmed our deep love for each other before he died. Yet my own nightmarish struggles with power and powerlessness continued. I had to be reconciled to the parts of myself I couldn't quite face. I had to differentiate the dream-image of my father from my actual father, and I had to differentiate my image of my father from my image of myself.

Reading Job's story, and his testimony of turmoil, I came to realize how much we had in common. What he processed was what I was processing. What he needed in his time, during his painful season, I needed in my time and my season. Job managed to deal with his own issues without allowing himself to be overtaken by his friends' distortions of the truth. Despite their pressures, he let himself give full vent to his anguish, his angst, his despair, and his disillusionment.

I found Job's example inspiring, even though I wasn't sure I was willing to go there in my own dialogue with God. Perhaps not so much because I didn't think God could handle it but because I worried about what I might find out about myself in the process. Did I dare open myself up that completely? Would I be able to live with the truth about myself? The therapist had told me from the onset that in the healing process, things get worse first before they get better. As I started to come to terms with the severity and plentitude of my internal conflicts, it was terrifying to consider. Frankly, I didn't want to go fishing in the abyss; I didn't want to know what monsters, what Leviathans, were swimming in the depths of the sea of my unconscious.

In the confrontation at the end of the story, the Lord challenged Job, "Can you draw out Leviathan with a fishhook, or press down its tongue with a cord?" (Job 41:1). He made it plain that this sea-monster (an archetypal image if ever there was one, and an image of the prince of darkness, the adversary) could not be tamed by anyone but God. Only its creator could handle it (see Job 41:7–11). I knew I couldn't do it. Yet I also knew the power of the monster swimming in my unconscious, waiting to devour me, depended on its being left alone in the deep, unnamed and unfaced. I also knew the prophetic promise: "On that day the LORD with his cruel and great and strong sword will punish Leviathan the fleeing serpent, Leviathan the twisting serpent, and he will kill the dragon that is in the sea" (Isaiah 27:1). That meant the time had come for me to catch it.

You might be exactly where I was. You might be as frightened as I was. But please know that the scariest place can also be your threshold. Step through it knowing you are not as alone as you think. God has not dropped you from His hands. He is at the threshold with you, and your healing can happen right in the middle of your chaos. Stick with Him. Walk straight through your uncertainty, unsettledness, and tears, knowing who is walking with you.

QUESTIONS TO PONDER

» What does it mean for you to be emotionally honest?

» What do you need to do to become more emotionally honest?

» How do you handle the skeptical thoughts that show up in your mind? Do you challenge them? resist them? question them? submit to them? What about the cynical thoughts? And the judgmental thoughts?

» What do you need to do to become more aware of how you perceive your reality?

12

Fear and Hope

Each of us must confront our own fears, must come face to face
with them. How we handle our fears will determine where we
go with the rest of our lives. To experience adventure or to be
limited by the fear of it.

Judy Blume, *Tiger Eyes*

One of the hardest things to learn is to give voice to your
pain while also differentiating between your voice and the
accuser's voice. Fear and hope often exist side by side. We see
hope as something good, but we must also realize that not all
fear is demonic. Some fears will keep you from making foolish choices and causing harm. What is important is to recognize what you fear and realize that not every thought is your
thought. Knowing the difference will make your hard seasons
more fruitful and easier to bear.

The final stanza of Job's initial poem includes one of the most familiar and misinterpreted passages in the book. How you interpret these few lines profoundly impacts how you interpret the whole of the story, including the outcomes at the end. Most of us aren't Hebrew scholars, but we need to note that this stanza is difficult if not impossible to translate. According to biblical studies and Hebrew scholar Francis Andersen, "The last three verses of Job's speech are so unintelligible in the Hebrew original that translators have had to take various liberties to secure reasonable English."[1] In other words, all our translations of this passage are approximations of what the Hebrew says. This is the way the NRSV renders Job 3:24–26:

> My sighing comes like my bread,
>   and my groanings are poured out like water.
> Truly the thing that I fear comes upon me,
>   and what I dread befalls me.
> I am not at ease, nor am I quiet;
>   I have no rest; but trouble comes.

This is the NKJV:

> My sighing comes before I eat,
>   And my groanings pour out like water.
> For the thing I greatly feared has come upon me,
>   And what I dreaded has happened to me.
> I am not at ease, nor am I quiet;
>   I have no rest, for trouble comes.

And this is from the NASB:

> My groaning comes at the sight of my food,
>   And my cries pour out like water.
> For what I fear comes upon me,
>   And what I dread encounters me.

I am not at ease, nor am I quiet,
And I am not at rest, but turmoil comes.

We need to approach this text carefully, not only because it's so difficult to translate but also because it deals with the most delicate of issues. We should be careful but not intimidated, because a good reading guided by the Spirit's wisdom in the work of God-loving scholars and the teachings of the great doctors of the faith will point us to Jesus, showing us something essential about what it means to live a Spirit-led, cross-shaped life.

Job begins by telling us that his "bread," what he is living on, are his sighings. Actually "sighing" isn't the best word for what the Hebrew indicates. This is the same word used when the king of Egypt died, and the sons of Israel were profoundly oppressed and discouraged: "After a long time the king of Egypt died. The Israelites groaned under their slavery and cried out. Out of the slavery their cry for help rose up to God" (Exodus 2:23). That word for "groan" is translated "sigh" in Job. Do you think the sons of Israel under the oppression of slavery in Egypt were merely "sighing"? Jeremiah, the weeping prophet, used this same word in Lamentations: "The roads to Zion mourn, for no one comes to the festivals; all her gates are desolate, her priests groan; her young girls grieve, and her lot is bitter" (1:4).

The people of Judah, Jeremiah's people, lost everything—their city with its walls and gates, and their Temple with its altars. They were now captives in Babylon as they once had been slaves in Egypt. The priests were not merely sighing, they were *groaning*.

David, struggling with grave illness, used the word as well: "My eyes waste away because of grief; they grow weak because of all my foes" (Psalm 6:7).

So, as I said, "sighing" doesn't quite convey the gravity or intensity of Job's pain. Scholar John Hartley explains that the

Hebrew term refers to "the loud moans or wails that arise from those doing oppressive, slave labor or from a people devastated by a tragedy"[2] That is what Job was feeding on in his ash heap: loud moans and wails! One translation of the passage uses the word *shrieks*, which is far more accurate. A psalmist also used the word in almost this exact sense: "Because of my loud groaning my bones cling to my skin" (Psalm 102:5). And this is not far from how Jesus cried out in His dereliction on the cross: "My God, My God, why . . ." As we know, those words are drawn from Psalm 22, which opens with this question: "Why are you so far from helping me, from the words of my groaning?" (verse 1).

According to the Gospels, as Jesus was suffering on the cross, as He was praying Psalm 22, He was also issuing loud cries, shrieks, and moans (see Matthew 27:46–50; Mark 15:34–37; Luke 23:46). We must not gloss over these details, however small they may seem at first. Extreme distress drives us to lift our voice in shrieks and moans. And the same happened with Jesus, who, as the Scripture says, was touched with the feeling of our infirmities. He knows what it means to be driven beyond our limits. He knows what it is not only to sigh but also to groan, to cry out, to shriek. Not only does He know what we go through, He also went through it Himself in order to make it known in a new way.

During parts of my worst season, I was so numb that I could not bring my pain to speech. I was also reluctant to open up the deep places in my soul, afraid the monsters lurking there might emerge to devour me. Eventually, however, the torment became unbearable. I finally gave myself permission to do what Job and David and Jeremiah and Jesus had done: cry out with all my force, holding nothing back.

Hear what I am saying! I had to give myself permission to give my pain voice. I had to find my voice in my pain! I had lost my voice in my pain, and the only way to get my voice back was to find it in there as well.

Job began his complaint with a death wish. He cursed the day he was born. Not that he was contemplating suicide, but he saw death as a blessing compared to the life he was now forced to live. Beloved, I want to say this so emphatically to you: If you are wrestling in the night, terrified by the realization that you prefer death to life, you are not alone! Others have been where you are and moved through it to the other side. Job was there. He preferred death to life. Yet he pressed forward, as difficult as that may have been, and in the end was vindicated by God for his faithfulness. There is always hope, *always*. Please never forget that.

How the Forces of Darkness Work

The enemy never fights fair. Whenever the saints despair of life, as Job did, and as Paul did, the accuser rushes in to demonize them with suicidal ideations. So let me speak directly and emphatically: If and when those thoughts show up, recognize them for what they are. They are not your own thoughts. They are the insinuations of evil, an assault by the powers of darkness on you in your weakened state.

No, you will not find anything about the demonic in the *Diagnostic and Statistical Manual of Mental Disorders*. The *DSM* deals strictly with the rational or natural, not the supernatural or mysterious. It is very useful for psychiatrists, clinical psychologists, and therapists, but it cannot talk to us about the reality of the satanic and demonic realms. Historically, the *DSM* has avoided the issue of the demonic altogether, and at times clinicians have considered any talk of the supernatural as delusional. There is some evidence now within the helping professions that such a posture may be changing for some, although certainly not for all.

Be that as it may, the Christian tradition beginning with Jesus has always affirmed the reality of an invisible world and the presence of evil entities. The greatest sages and saints throughout the ages have borne witness to the reality of spiritual warfare in their lives, confirming the teaching of Scripture. And Scripture's teaching is abundantly clear: We have an enemy that marshals hordes of demonic spirits against us to hinder, annoy, harass, and oppress. Even so, we will fail to discern rightly what is happening so long as we lack an understanding of how the powers of darkness work. Remember Paul's warning:

> Anyone whom you forgive, I also forgive. What I have forgiven, if I have forgiven anything, has been for your sake in the presence of Christ. And we do this so that we may not be outwitted by Satan; for we are not ignorant of his designs.
>
> 2 Corinthians 2:10–11

The word for "designs" can also be translated "schemes" and implies "the content of thinking and reasoning."[3] It suggests that the enemy works on us by affecting our thinking, and we're most vulnerable when we're unaware that he works this way. So it's important to remember that all our thoughts "come" to us. Discerning where they come from matters immensely. Not all our thoughts come from us; some come from our heart and others don't. These other thoughts "come" in a similar fashion to the thoughts of our heart, yet they are sourced in our enemy's lies, planted in our minds by the evil one.

When I gave voice to my worst thoughts, Vinnie often reminded me: "Those thoughts aren't your personality; they are your enemy." That was sound spiritual advice. And my therapist often reminded me of a related truth: "You are not your thoughts." This difference is crucial. Accepting that certain thoughts have come to you is altogether different from welcoming them or believing they are yours. One of the ways we frustrate the enemy is by refusing to "own" the thoughts he tries to implant in our minds.

Paul used a different word in Ephesians to describe the ways in which the powers of darkness work: "Put on the whole armor of God, so that you may be able to stand against the wiles of the devil" (6:11). That word, *wiles*,[4] is tied to methods and strategies, which speaks to the fact that the powers of darkness devise schemes to afflict and trouble us, seeking to deepen our pain, diminish our well-being, and devastate our lives.

No, there is not a demon lurking behind every corner. But to ignore the reality of evil is dangerously naïve. Again, the forces of darkness never fight fair. They prey on our vulnerabilities and susceptibilities to temptations, taking advantage of our internal issues, unfinished business, defense mechanisms, and avoidance strategies whenever they can.

The "gates of Hades," as T. Austin-Sparks once said, are "the councils . . . of hell,"[5] which are the councils of death itself. Consider these words of David:

> Lift up your heads, O gates! and be lifted up, O ancient doors! that the King of glory may come in. Who is the King of glory? The Lord, strong and mighty, the Lord, mighty in battle. Lift up your heads, O gates! and be lifted up, O ancient doors! that the King of glory may come in. Who is this King of glory? The Lord of hosts, he is the King of glory.
>
> Psalm 24:7–11

At one level, this refers to Christ's triumphant ascension into heaven as the God-Man; having disarmed the principalities and powers, He now enters His glory with the spoils of battle. The doors and gates of Jerusalem, the Holy City, were indeed ancient. Yet there are other doors, equally real and even more ancient: the gates of hell itself. Christ, we confess, descended into hell, and plundered the darkness, taking the keys of death, hell, and the grave from the prince of darkness. So, Austin-Sparks argues:

> There are other doors mentioned in this connection beside the Everlasting doors. There are "The gates of Hades," which means the councils and schemes and judgments of hell. These are represented as being against the Church. It is therefore said that, because of the heavenly union with and in Him who has passed triumphantly through the everlasting doors, these other "gates" shall not prevail, because His sovereignty is in the Church and the Church is in His Sovereignty.[6]

Much as the United Nations Security Council gathers in New York City for their weighty business, and much as the angelic majesties and those appointed from the saints who have gone before us gather in the presence of the Triune God to deliberate on behalf of the Church, so too hell has a council.[7] The demonic hordes under the dominion of the prince of darkness craft schemes to oppose the work God is doing in His people. Their goal, as we know, is to bring death and destruction, to corrupt, to deceive and delude. We are not to be ignorant of that. We are, as Jesus made clear, to "keep awake and pray" so we "may not come into the time of trial" (Mark 14:38).[8]

The trial Jesus warned the disciples about is the one the enemy wants to inflict. Its diabolical purpose is to make the faithful fall. The trial of God, however, has another purpose, a divine purpose. When God puts us to the test, it is never for the purpose of causing us to fall. So when we consider the dialogue in the opening chapters of Job that takes place between Yahweh and the Satan, we need to bear in mind that God is not the servant.

We also need to bear in mind that God is not in any way, shape, or form the cause of evil. The devil is God's enemy as well as ours; he accuses God just as he accuses the saints. The enemy is neither omnipotent nor omniscient nor omnipresent.

He spends his time wandering to and fro on the earth. The Sovereign Lord, by contrast, is omnipresent, omniscient, and omnipotent! He is God all by Himself. And He is good. God is not only *not* the author or the cause of evil, but He cannot even be tempted to do anything evil (see James 1:13). That means that when God chooses to prove someone, it is always for their good and His glory. Our God causes all things to work together for those who love Him and are the called according to His purpose (see Romans 8:28).

So while it may appear that the adversary was provoking God to do something sinister against Job, that wasn't even in God's mind. God loved Job with an everlasting love and already knew Job inside out, better than Job knew himself. All that He allowed was for Job's vindication, the defeat of Job's enemy, and the salvation of Job's friends. Likewise, whatever difficulty He allows you to endure will ultimately serve His purposes and your well-being.

God Is a Good God and the Devil Is . . .

We desperately need to learn to read the Sacred Text faithfully, and that requires us to read the biblical texts as they are intended to be read. Job is an epic poem, a long riddle that needs to be solved. It is shot through with profound and troubling questions, and when all is said and done, it provides us with anything but nice, tidy answers. While this should be obvious, for many it is not: Poetry, including biblical poetry, cannot be read the way a romance novel or even a medical report is read. Poetry takes a different slant on human experience, invites expression of emotions and feelings, and stretches the imagination with well-chosen metaphors. To ignore the literary style of Job is to miss the whole point.

Within the canon, the book of Job belongs to the Wisdom Literature of the Old Testament, alongside Psalms, Proverbs,

Ecclesiastes, and the Song of Solomon (also known as Song of Songs). The wisdom tradition seeks to know where wisdom can be found. Job raised that very question himself in the heart of his complaint: "Where shall wisdom be found? And where is the place of understanding?" (Job 28:12). He argued that human beings cannot find the path of wisdom because it cannot be found either in the land of the living or the realm of death. God alone understands the path to wisdom. God alone knows its place. So the conclusion Job drew was the same as the one Solomon and his father, David, drew: "The fear of the Lord, that is wisdom; and to depart from evil is understanding" (Job 28:28). That tells us that Job is a riddle intended to teach us the fear of the Lord. We have to bear that in mind as we consider the conversation in the chambers of heaven between the Lord and the adversary.

Clearly, the accuser is powerful and should not be taken lightly. But we need to remember that he is granted those powers and uses them only as he is allowed to use them. He is simply no match for the almighty God. We also need to remember that God is not only all-powerful but also wholly good. When all hell breaks loose in our lives, we may feel God has abandoned us, leaving us at the mercy of the prince of darkness. Yet if we are familiar with the whole counsel of God and intimate with the body of wisdom revealed in the sacred Scriptures, we will stand fast in the knowledge of God's power and goodness. Whatever the enemy is doing is not what God is doing, and what God is doing is infinitely greater. The enemy always means what he does for evil. God always means what He does for good.

The late Morris Cerullo, whom I cherished as a friend and considered a father of the Pentecostal heritage, would often say in his preaching, tongue-in-cheek and with a twinkle in his eye, "I have a deep revelation. Are you ready?" He would then pause to draw us in, preparing us to ponder what he was about to say, which was: "God is a good God! And the devil is a bad devil!" His statement and the way he delivered it might make you chuckle, but it is utterly brilliant, theologically and psychologically. You can't just happen on that conclusion based on a cursory review of the Scriptures. You must live a life of profound faith, wrestling with the Sacred Text and the ancient teachings of the faith in order to be able to say what Morris Cerullo said. Indeed, God is a good God, and the devil is a bad devil.

We always begin with the premise that God is good. He can be nothing but good. God in His very essence is immeasurable goodness. He is goodness personified. His goodness is so great that I cannot comprehend it fully. I can only know that God brings me to those very places of transformation in my life that I need to be taken to. Not only is God immeasurably good, He is also infinite and perfect love. God never wills evil for any of His children. As a matter of fact, He never wills evil for any human being. As the Scripture says, it is not God's will that any should perish; it is His will that all come to repentance (see 2 Peter 3:9). Whether they do or not is not God's decision, because God's sovereignty is that of a loving parent, not that of a tyrannical monarch.[9]

If you hear nothing else from me in this entire self-disclosure, hear this: My fears of God being more judge than lover caused me great harm, due in part to my sense of my own profound flaws and failures. Yet in my dark season I came to know Him in fresh ways, ways new to me but in fact ancient. I came to know His healing as I'd never been able to understand it before. And in that process, I learned to honor the ancient faith and the teachings of the early doctors of the Church. Since that season, I often say: "Out with the old and in with the older!"

God is love. Make no mistake about that. Yes, He is Judge. Yet to comprehend Him as Judge we must look to the slain

Lamb and how He judges. The bottom line is that the power God exercises is one of love. And God is not a dysfunctional parent.

If that is true, what are we to make of Job's statement, oft cited by so-called faith teachers: "Truly the thing that I fear comes upon me, and what I dread befalls me" (Job 3:25)? Does this mean Job created his own troubles through something like the so-called "law of attraction"? In a word, no. I know that's a popular interpretation and I don't want to be uncharitable, but I do want to be abundantly clear: Such thinking, however "deep" it may sound to some, is wholly at odds with the mind of the Spirit and the teaching of the Scriptures. It is profoundly dangerous to tell people they're to blame for their own pain because they allowed themselves to be afraid! That misrepresents the character of God, misleads the untaught, and further damages those who are already hurting.

Even if, for the sake of argument, we assume that what Job suffered had something to do with his fear, we first must ask ourselves this question: If God is all-powerful and perfectly loving—and He has revealed Himself to be exactly that in the death and resurrection of Jesus Christ—then what would be the purpose in allowing Job to experience all the results of his fearful apprehensions? The only sound answer we might give is that Job was able to see that no matter what befell him in life, absolutely nothing could separate him from God's love. In other words, if Job's fear was a factor at all in what happened, it was only because God wanted to deliver him from it. This cannot be argued any other way. To do so is to malign the testimony of Holy Writ and the very character and nature of the God and Father of our Lord Jesus Christ.

All that said, Job's torments were severe. Within his complaint, Job took a mental journey to the abode of the dead. He imagined those who were shut up in Sheol. In his day, kings were buried with their treasures in hopes that this wealth would bring them comfort in the afterlife. Yet what of those whose lives had been bitter and empty? Job argued that he would not find torment but rather peace because even the wicked no longer had anyone to trouble them after death. Those who had been oppressed were no longer disturbed. They no longer had to hear the voice of their oppressors. Death, in other words, was the great equalizer for Job.

Whether one is small or great, whether one is wealthy or poor, death is a relief, a release from all pain. Hence, at this point, Job declared he would prefer death to life—and understandably so. He suffered the loss of all his property, his goods, his children, and his health. He lost the support of his friends and perhaps the companionship of his wife. Worst, he lost the comfort of what he thought he knew about God and about his relation to God. When you have finally lost everything that matters in your life, what good is your life to you?

It would be a mistake to think Job suffered from what today we would call a psychological disorder (such as obsessive-compulsive disorder or generalized anxiety disorder). All parents are concerned about their children. We don't know that Job was *continually* apprehensive about his children's relationship to God. If his concern drove an obsessive offering of sacrifices on their behalf, that would indicate profound instability and uncertainty in his relationship to God, his family, and his own identity and personhood. Yet based on what God said of him and what he said about himself and about God, we see that was not the case.

When you carefully read Job's complaint and his defense of his integrity, there's a genuine sense of mental clarity, an absence of anything obsessive or overwhelming, no signs of a cognitive disorder (such as extreme anxiety or inordinate and extreme fear). Job simply doesn't present that kind of symptomatology in his self-disclosure.

Let's consider the question from a different angle. What else might Job mean by his confession, "The thing that I fear comes upon me"? Why might the Spirit have given this complaint to us in inspired Scripture? First and foremost, Job was very clear that the dread he felt in his mind and his body profoundly impacted him. That is not only understandable but to be expected. Today we would say that the losses he endured traumatized him; we would diagnose him as suffering from post-traumatic stress disorder (PTSD). Those who survive a natural disaster or live through a terrorist act experience a similar kind of dread. They suffer deeply intense and disturbing thoughts and feelings long after the traumatic event is over. Knowing someone who had suffered in that way, would you, in the name of God, tell them that their fears had created all their troubles? To do so would be cruel and accusatory, would it not? Nothing good comes of blaming victims or accusing them of bringing disaster down on their own heads. That thinking has nothing to do with the truth, and it bears all the marks of what James calls demonic wisdom (see James 3:14–16).

Notice, too, that when Job spoke of his fear, he did so in the present tense. Don't be deceived by the fact that in some English translations it is rendered in the past tense; it implies present-tense dread. Job also told us what came from this ongoing dread: "I am not at ease, nor am I quiet; I have no rest; but trouble comes" (Job 3:26). None of this is past tense in the Hebrew; it is present-tense reality. Job felt totally helpless, utterly powerless, incapable of taking rest or being at peace even for a moment. Given what we now know about trauma, it is evident that he was processing the aftereffects of the shock of his ordeal. He had been traumatized, left utterly restless and without peace. I can relate because that is where I found myself in my dark season. And I can tell you that if it had not been for the grace of God, I would never have survived.

I can also tell you this beyond any shadow of a doubt: While I certainly had to face my fears and recognize how they were preventing me from fully enjoying the love of God, those fears did not create the troubles that converged and hit me like a bus. Whatever their influence on my well-being, my fears had absolutely no control over other people's decisions. My fears didn't create the financial and legal challenges our church faced. My fears didn't corrupt our deliberations during the discernment process or the great caution I exercised. What happened in my life was a "wild card" or "black swan" event.[10] Such events are extremely rare and cannot be anticipated. So, again, even if Job's fears were unfounded, they were not in any way to blame for what happened to him or his children or his livestock. His troubles were so vast, so complex, and so malevolent that he could not have anticipated them at all. What was true for him was true for me, and at times it will be true for you!

Stephen Hooks, in his commentary on Job, explained how exceptional Job's experience was, and why he was allowed to suffer what he suffered:

> First . . . God does not ordinarily act this way towards his servants. God's affliction of Job is not to be understood as the norm. Second, God says that the Satan incited me against him. This point, too, is crucial to our understanding of Job's struggle. Though the Satan may have encouraged and even carried out the affliction of Job (cf. v. 7), it was God who actually authorized it. With these words Yahweh accepts responsibility for Job's suffering, and it is from Yahweh that Job seeks deliverance in the dialogue. Third, God characterizes his ruin of Job as without any cause. This finally establishes the very point on which the dialogue turns and which the book on the whole is written to address—Job has done nothing to deserve the suffering that has befallen him. God does not always operate on a principle of retribution. In his management of his world, he

does not always see to it that people get what they deserve. Life, as God presides over it, is not always just.[11]

If we read the story of Job rightly, remembering that it is a poem and a riddle that belongs to the Wisdom Literature, we recognize that Job's suffering is outsized and extreme. What happened to him is more intense and extensive than what happens to anyone else, apart from Jesus. Anyone who endured even a third of what Job endured would be overwhelmed by it. But the exception proves the rule.

The Spirit has given us Job's story as inspired Scripture to teach us many things, not least of which is that we have an enemy who seeks to destroy us. Job's story reveals that evil is powerful and its effects are exceedingly difficult to deal with in this fallen world. But Job's story also reveals that we can trust ourselves absolutely to the goodness and power of the God who loves us perfectly. When we read Job's story faithfully, we receive the same comfort offered by the aged apostle John in his first letter to his community: "Little children, you are from God, and have conquered . . . for the one who is in you is greater than the one who is in the world" (1 John 4:4). The mystery of iniquity is indeed a mystery. But the mystery of the Triune God revealed in the death of Jesus Christ is infinitely greater.

QUESTIONS TO PONDER

» In what specific ways is fear creating stress in your life? What about anger? Are there any lingering fears you have had to deal with since you were a child?

» How do you feel about yourself in relation to the fears you wrestle with, and how have you coped with those fears?

» For you, is God more Lover or Judge? Precisely how do you see God as Lover? as Judge?

» When has it been safe for you to be totally honest with God?

Epilogue

Daring to Dream

The disadvantages and dangers of the author's calling are offset by an advantage so great as to make all its difficulties, disappointments, and maybe hardships, unimportant. . . . Nothing befalls him that he cannot transmute into a stanza, a song, or a story, and having done this, be rid of it. The artist is the only free man.

W. Somerset Maugham, *The Summing Up*

I have taken great care in putting into words, the best I can, aspects of my personal journey through a profoundly traumatic season. I realize that it is impossible to do justice to the many complexities I faced and learned from. In dealing with my memories, I had to take time to reflect on certain aspects of the experience that have left an indelible mark on my psyche. And I did it knowing that we live in a world where formulas and quick-fix techniques are more popular than truthful wrestling with the profoundly complex dynamics of the human condition.

I tried to write this book in a way that is congruent with how I lived through the season I've described. I've returned to many of the same themes in these chapters, considering those themes from slightly different perspectives and angles. I did that because in my difficult season I had to recycle again and again through various memories, plumbing the depths of the way God has made me. Not only did I have to come to terms with my experiences again and again, I had to come to terms with how I responded to them or reacted against them.

The student in me, the one who desires to love God with his mind as well as his heart, has known for a long time that all truth is God's truth, even if some of God's servants would prefer that not to be the case. The Church would not be where it is in its understanding of the truth if the likes of Irenaeus, Tertullian, the Cappadocian Fathers, Athanasius, and Augustine had ignored interdisciplinary studies of philosophy, metaphysics, physics, cosmology, etc. We would be foolish to think that Jesus and His apostles were unaware of the works of Greek philosophers and the various schools of thought in the ancient world.

The same holds for the rabbis, as one glance at the work of Philo in the first century shows. The apostle Paul was schooled by Gamaliel and a graduate of the university of Tarsus. He would have been considered one of the great scholars of his day. Sadly, many in our circles have an aversion to any education other than that which comes through the individual's devotional study of Scripture. But that aversion has nothing to do with the Holy Spirit. Rather, it is the conditioning of a culture that has learned to question every authority except the authority of one's own opinion. And it erodes our ability to do theology faithfully or engage the Sacred Text with sound methodologies of interpretation.

The work of psychology dates far back in history, and careful study of the ancient Church reveals that the Patristics were deeply concerned with the cure of the human soul, the human psyche, and the human being. Certainly, from the nineteenth century on, beginning with Freud, whose theories for the most part have been dismissed by even the psychological community, you could say that a distrust of all things psychological had some validity. The challenge is that since that time, and more particularly in the last century, the integration of long-term studies on the life cycle, the adult life span, the behavior of children, family systems, coupling systems, and community systems can only be ignored out of pure judgmentalism, and ultimately to our own detriment. Many advances in the world of therapeutic consciousness also have served us well. Those who are willing to do the work of integrating the theological and the psychological, giving themselves to careful study, will be expertly equipped to come alongside the people of God to help guide their way into peace. I know some will find fault with portions of what I have written, if not all of it. But I'm not writing for my opponents. I'm writing for the struggling, distressed, downcast, despairing, anxious, and traumatized saints who have grown disillusioned by the flat and trite answers offered by those who have not done the work necessary to speak with knowledge and understanding.

I am equally aware that there are those within Christian circles who will find fault with the emphasis I place on satanic and demonic reality and activity. Again, while I understand that there have been many abuses and excesses in relation to understanding and dealing with the realms of the satanic and demonic, to dismiss them as merely the product of an unenlightened ancient Near Eastern culture is hubris of the worst sort. I make no apologies either to those who deny the work of the demonic, or to those who wish to explain it away as mythological. My purpose in this book is neither to provide a detailed exegesis nor to combat exegetical fallacies. My purpose is only to reach to the core of the hearts of those who know what it is to be personally oppressed by evil powers.

Having said that, for you who have derived some benefit from my self-disclosure, please know that the best I can do is share only what I know. I do not have all the answers. My only claim is that what I know has changed my life, and I know *who* has changed my life! It is His grace that I commend to you, and His power that I attest to for your sake.

The House I Lived In

They say hindsight is 20/20. That may not be the whole truth, but it does seem that the more we reflect on where we have been, the more we learn about what we went through and what resulted from it. That is certainly the case for me. And I want to close this book by fully unpacking the dream I shared with you earlier, the one that came to me in the earliest part of my dark season. First, though, I need to set the stage by giving you a bit more of my history in that house.

It was, as I said, my paternal grandparents' house. In the main, it was for me a place of great comfort and safety. I am not saying our family was perfect. We had issues, sorrows, pains, and sins to deal with (though we surely did not deal with them all). Despite our dysfunction, however, the entire extended family was in church every Sunday morning. My great-uncle on my mother's side of the family established the first Italian Protestant Chapel in New York City at the turn of the twentieth century for the sake of Italian-speaking immigrants who lived on Staten Island. Within not too many years, that one chapel became three campuses spread apart to account for the many who sought solace in hearing the gospel.

While the stereotype held that all Italians are Catholic, my great-uncle was Protestant and was also fruitful in sharing the love of Jesus with Catholics. He did so in a simple way with simple folk who required simple faith. He was seminary trained, and well-versed in the many ways in which the Scriptures were being challenged by Enlightenment thinking. Yet he held to his conviction that the Scripture was holy and true.

As it turned out, my parents met at church and eventually were married there. My father was the church organist and choir director. The services were arranged to give my father the time to ride his bicycle from campus to campus to play for the worship services and direct all the choirs.

As the church grew, it attracted an English-speaking audience. The church began to hold services both in Italian and in English. Uncle Frank brought in another pastor to handle the English-speaking crowd, though he too was Italian. Years later, when Uncle Frank retired, he assumed the full leadership of the church. Most of those who were attracted to the English-speaking services were considered by others as the marginalized, the disenfranchised, the excluded, and the unwelcomed.

By the time I was growing up, those three campuses belonged to the Presbyterian Synod of New York City and the Presbyterian Church of America. I worshiped every Sunday in a congregation filled with Italian and Irish immigrants, African Americans, Hispanic Americans, and various other ethnic groups. I didn't realize then that Providence had His hand on me, nor did I understand how those circumstances that formed and shaped me from my birth would determine the trajectory of my life and ministry.

Grandma and Grandpa bought a house that became the center of our entire extended Chironna family for three generations. They lived there and held the space for us until my grandmother, who outlived Grandpa, died at about ninety-six years of age. At times growing up in that house reminded me of the line from Charles Dickens's *A Tale of Two Cities*: "It was the best of times, it was the worst of times." Yet even amid our family's heartaches, economic hardships, intense arguments, and seasons of separation, we experienced pristine moments in which the profound sense of love, harmony, joy, and deep gladness provided relief.

I loved Grandma and Grandpa, and they loved me and all of my cousins. They enjoyed our company. They enjoyed having us in one house. And we enjoyed living with them. I was allowed to go to bed a little late, so I would often come downstairs from the second floor, where I lived with Mom and Dad, to sit on the floor beside Grandpa while he kicked back in his favorite easy chair, his feet up on the ottoman. Some nights I watched television with him, shows now considered classics: *Gunsmoke, Wagon Train, Maverick, Bat Masterson, Fury*, and *The Rifleman*. Even now, as I give it thought, it moves me to tears. Grandpa made me feel safe! Grandma did, too, for that matter.

It's not that my parents didn't make me feel safe, but at that time in my life, my dad was doing his best to run the family business, which required a great deal of energy and time and put him under a lot of stress. Mom worked as the bookkeeper, and that required much of her time. Even as a child, I knew the price they were paying to give me the best life possible. Yet the times with Grandma and Grandpa were especially seminal. To this day, I'm a diehard New York Yankees fan, probably because every Saturday Grandpa turned his little black-and-white wicker-cabinet television set to the game. We watched Mickey Mantle, Roger Maris, Elston Howard, and many other greats! Fun as they were to watch, it was equally fun to see Grandpa's excitement when they took the lead and won.

The big family gatherings were always in the basement. In those days, unless you had lots of money, which our families did not, the basements were not fully finished. That basement holds so many memories for me. If you came into the house from the side doorway in the back, you could walk up a short flight of stairs to the first floor where Grandma and Grandpa lived or you could take a left turn at the top of that short flight, following the staircase up to the second floor where Dad, Mom, and I lived. But if you entered by another door, you would find a longer flight of stairs, flanked on both sides by Sheetrock and a certain kind of wood paneling dating back to the 1930s. From the top of those stairs, you could see the basement floor, which was smoothed concrete, darkened and gray from use. As you reached the bottom stair and stepped onto the floor, the entire basement opened up. To the left behind the stairwell wall was a large table that seated twenty people, leaving space at the far end for people to walk. On that far wall was Grandpa's icebox, which he kept stocked with soda and other beverages. There were three windows at street level: one where Grandpa and Grandma sat at the head of the table; one on the far wall that looked out onto the patio in the backyard; and one above the icebox with a view across Grandpa's tomato garden and into the neighbor's house.

Directly in front of me, standing at the bottom of the stairs and facing the back wall, was a green Formica kitchen table that could seat eight. When dinner was just a few of us, Grandpa would sit on the end of the table to the right and Grandma on the end to the left. On the far wall behind the table was a big porcelain double sink. Grandma did a lot of her cleaning and preparing at that sink. To the right of the sink was a large stove, which she used for all our large gatherings, as well as our Thursday night meals. To the immediate right of the stove a large sheet had been strung up to cover the doorway to a makeshift pantry. In the floor under the curtain, there was a drain used for wastes like hot oils and grease. Behind that curtain were Grandma's canned goods, pastas, spices, and crates of soda, as well as anything and everything else Grandma might need for the meals she made for us.

Looking to my right, still standing at the foot of the stairs, I could see the doorway that stood about fifteen feet ahead of me. A hanging sheet served as a makeshift door, marking the transition into the back of the basement. In that room was a single lightbulb, a large fuel-oil furnace, and shelves of canned goods. Way back on the far wall was an old porcelain tub. About three feet to its left was an old oak barrel. A long, thin, dark brown plastic tube ran from the barrel into the drain in the bottom of the tub.

Remember, my grandparents were Italian immigrants, and like virtually all Italian immigrants at that time, they grew grapes in the backyard. When the grapes ripened, they gathered them, washed them, and poured them into the bathtub. Then Grandma and Grandpa got in their stocking feet and crushed those grapes, starting the process of making their homemade wine. Behind the bathtub was a portion of the first concrete wall that separated the beginning of the porch in the front of the house from the back of the porch. It had been broken through in a less-than-perfect way to give enough room for Grandpa to store his tools in the dirt under the porch. The hole in the wall was big enough for him to crawl in on all fours to grab his tools as he needed them.

Closer to the doorway that led to the back of the basement, just beyond the wall of the stairwell, was a spare bed and a chest of drawers. It was kept in a large cubbyhole between the stairwell wall and the Sheetrock wall that separated the front of the basement from the back of the basement where the furnace, the jarred goods, the porcelain tub, the oak barrel, and Grandpa's tools were. At the head of the bed was another window at street level where you could see, from below, Grandpa's car parked in the driveway. Uncle Vito lived in Manhattan, and every few weekends he would come to Staten Island to spend time with the family. He slept on that spare bed and put his clothes in that chest of drawers.

As I mentioned, in that back part of the basement where the furnace was, there was a single incandescent lightbulb hanging by a wire from a rafter. Turning it on or off required pulling a long string attached to the switch. The sheet hanging over the doorway kept that space especially dark, so none of us kids wanted to venture back there, at least when the adults were not around. Who knew what was lurking in the dark? Like most little kids, we avoided the dark like a plague. We preferred to play in the basement with light streaming in from all the windows.

Now, back to the dream.

From a Nightmare to a Dream

I am standing outside the back entrance to my grandparents' house. It's dark and foreboding. I'm not sure if it's evening or morning. I know the house is totally empty, because no one lives there anymore. The door is open. I feel that I'm supposed to go in. I would have preferred to go up the short flight of stairs to Grandma and Grandpa's floor or at least to continue up the winding staircase to Mom and Dad's rooms. But I know I'm not allowed.

I enter and descend the staircase. Somehow, I see the dark, smooth floor below me, though no lights are on. I am descending into the dark. At the bottom of the stairwell, I stand, as I know I must, assessing what I see. To my left is the large family table. On the far wall is Grandpa's icebox. Immediately in front of me is the smaller kitchen table with its several chairs. Behind it are the old porcelain sink and the old stove. To the right of that are the Sheetrock wall and the pantry doorway covered with an old sheet. Farther ahead is the doorway to the back of the house, the furnace room. I feel I need to walk toward it. As I do, I pass the spare bed Uncle Vito slept in and the chest of drawers he used. The windows aren't allowing much light in, as it is dark and overcast outside.

Now comes the moment I've dreaded. I must pull back the curtain that covers the darkest, dingiest part of the basement, the room my cousins and I avoided when we were alone. I pull back the curtain, and something unexpected happens. In the barest, slightest light, which is coming from who knows where,

I see on the far end another door with another sheet, a dim light showing around its edges.

I recognize this is a change, as this door had not been there in our house. Nonetheless, I feel I have to face whatever is behind this unexpected door. The dread and suspense I feel are palpable. I break out in a cold sweat. I find the courage to pull back the sheet and enter. Lo and behold, I am not in the basement anymore. I am standing in a graveyard.

In Charles Dickens's novella *A Christmas Carol*, the Ghost of Christmas Future takes Ebenezer Scrooge to a graveyard and shows him his own grave. I'm now standing in a similar scene. I cannot explain how I know, but I am somewhere in northern Europe in what I take to be the United Kingdom. The trees around me are all dark and barren, the sky overcast. Directly before me is a gravestone, a massive one, slightly uprooted from the ground, tilted from the eroding and shifting of the earth over centuries and centuries. It is made of granite and oxidized with a green patina. This graveyard has been here a long, long time. Whoever is buried under this gravestone has been dead a long, long time. The dark leafless branches of huge trees bending over the graveyard seem ominous.

The entire scene is eerie, even terrifying. I'm frozen and cannot move. I recognize the aged, patinaed gravestone as an ancient Celtic cross, though it looks exactly like the Presbyterian cross I remember from the church of my youth. I don't at all like the feelings I experience as I stand here. I don't like them at all. I'm troubled and perplexed. Then I wake up.

This dream occurred not long after the bus ran me over. I shared it with the therapist. As a clinical psychologist, he was trained in dream interpretation and had helped me with other dreams. But he knew somehow this was one dream he should not touch. I now understand why. It has taken me years to sort it out. I did not know what to make of it at the time, and even what I thought I knew about it I did not understand very well.

But in hindsight, after much reflection, I can see that this dream contained the entire story of my dark season, and the promise that the season would end with a new level of freedom and a heightened sense of God's keeping power. It was assuring me that I would come out on the other side with greater clarity and insight into the anxiety and depression I had endured.

I have studied dreams, dreaming, and dream interpretation for decades from the perspective of three different disciplines: Scripture, theology, and psychology. I have read widely in the history of dream interpretation, including the history of Christian interpretation, and I have engaged at some level in the findings of neurological studies. In all of that, I have learned that dreams are a means for the unconscious to bring stability and clarity to every area of our being.

I have also learned that there are a multitude of approaches to dream interpretation. Those in the various disciplines who have studied dreams and dreaming have shown again and again that more often than not a dream is speaking to us about ourselves, even when we're dreaming about someone else.

I'm reticent to impose an interpretation on a dream, including a dream of my own. With all I've learned, I feel I still have much to learn. I know I have to respect the mystery of the dream, to take my time with it, to ask tons of questions about it, and to consider those questions and their possible answers from various angles before attempting an interpretation. In popular prophetic circles many are quick to claim frequent prophetic dreams. Yet in truth, very few dreams are prophetic. We're confused about that because we tend to interpret dreams as we interpret Scripture. Void of any real understanding, we rush to judgment, quickly leaping to the conclusions that confirm our biases. Worse, we're convinced that such quick judgments are a sign that God has given them to us.

I don't say this to shame anyone. I say this to invite us to a level of humility. We need to deal much more carefully with our dreams. We need to take pains to learn more appropriate ways of interpreting them. If we do not refuse simplicities and foolishness, we'll never learn the wisdom necessary for making good sense of our dreams. Remember, Joseph had to live with his dream thirteen years before he was able to fully understand what it meant!

It's taken me years to come to terms with what this dream means for me and why it came to me when it did. It was indeed a good dream, although I experienced it more as a nightmare. It located me in four domains. First, it placed me in my past, my origins—where I'd come from. Second, it located me in my present, my personhood—where I was. Third, it held me in the unknown, the mysterious—where I'd never been. Fourth, it located me in my future, my purpose—where I'd eventually be going.

At the time of the dream, the pain I was experiencing was excruciating psychologically and emotionally, as well as physically. I felt lost; I did not know whether I was coming or going. I had no sense of purpose, no direction home. The dream let me know I had to go back to the earliest stages of my life in my spirit, descending into that place in my heart where my will, my spirit, had been formed.

God Moves in Mysterious Ways

Much of my formation occurred in that house on 214 Bement Avenue. Even now, I know it like the back of my hand. So many of the memories stored deepest in my heart were made in that place. Yet in this dream, which came at the beginning of my season of trauma and terror, the place I'd always remembered as a haven of peace and safety filled me with dread. There was so much familiar to me in that house. Yet in the dream I was standing afraid, discovering that I had to face something unfamiliar, something unexpected in the one place I thought I knew so well. Why? Because our fears often present themselves to us to teach us how little we understand about what we think we know best. The closer we get to the truth, the more we resist it. (You might want to read that again).

To pass into the unexpected new, I had to cross the threshold of the old and familiar. That was the occasion of my dread. Life, real life, requires growth. And we can have no growth without crossing thresholds. That crossing always requires us to step through anxiety. To borrow from the imagery of Marcus Aurelius in his work *Meditations*, the descent down those stairs in my dream was a trip into the dark depths of my own inner house. The Lord was taking me into my deep basement, the darkest, dingiest places in my own history. He did not do this to destroy me but to free and to heal me. The Lord used that old ghost of the fear of the dark as a parable for me, a riddle to be solved. He did it so I could get past all the stuff I thought I knew to what was lurking in the dark, if indeed anything was.

Beloved, none of us knows our own depths. Only God knows. That is why David cries out, "Search me, O God, and know my heart; try me and know my anxious thoughts; and see if there be any hurtful way in me, and lead me in the everlasting way" (Psalm 139:23–24 NASB1995). David knew not to analyze himself, not to go down on his own into the depths of his heart. Whatever monsters lurked there, whatever fears, he knew he could not search them out. So he wisely cried out to God, asking God to do the searching. Sometimes, as in my case, God begins that searching by giving us dreams that take us back to the familiar, the already known, making it possible for us to know it all differently.

What the devil is up to and what God is up to are two entirely different things. What God does, God always means for good. The dream, in God's intention, was not to threaten or frighten me, or even to force me to face my fears. The anxiety I felt in the dream represented the effects of the trauma I had experienced when the bus ran me over. By calling me to overcome that anxiety by lifting the sheet and crossing the threshold into an unknown space, I was learning that I did not have to be afraid. The spirit that had terrorized me needed to be faced down, and for that confrontation I needed courage. The challenge was, I had been left in a weakened state by what I had suffered. I was depleted by the stress, and overwhelmed by the grief. So God allowed me to act out that courage in a dream, empowering me to do it when I was awake.

Standing at the bottom of the stairs, with my feet on the smooth concrete, I was at my lowest point. Around me were mementos of the past I'd shared with my family. The kitchen table was now empty, the light dimmer, the sink far more worn. I knew I had to turn away from all of that and walk across the threshold into that room I'd always avoided. Like Moses in the wilderness, who at the point farthest from his call had to turn aside toward the burning bush, I had to make a conscious choice to move in a different direction, to cross a threshold into the strange and unknown.

Metanoia is the Greek word we translate as "repentance." We've somehow turned it into a negative word. I've heard it used all too often in condemning ways. The call to repentance, however, is a call forward, not back. It is a matter of facing a different direction, a matter of changing perspectives, a matter of standing in new light so we can see what we have been missing all along.

Once I had pulled back the veil, I was standing on foreign soil. The dark dead branches of a massive tree loomed large over the grave and its gravestone. Everything around me spoke of death. It was a winter season; the skies were darkened, the tree barren. The date on the gravestone was mysterious and, in some ways, dreadful, although not at all diabolical. What did this cross mark? It marked the place of death. Up to that point I had not in my life fully faced my own mortality. But suddenly I found myself feeling and thinking that my life was over. My trauma threw me up against the ultimate limit of my existence. In the dream, I was facing the final enemy, standing eye to eye with my limits.

After I woke from the dream, I had to know where this grave was and what this cross was. I soon discovered that the cross was an ancient Celtic cross.[1] What did it symbolize? What I was facing in that dream was not only my own past but something far older. I know now God was drawing on my memories to bring me back not only to the faith of my youth but to the faith of the fathers, the ancient faith, the great tradition. Through the dream, the Lord was telling me that the way into my future lay not only through my past but through the past of the Church, and that the way into life lay through my share in Christ's death. To be crucified with Him is to live eternal life.

Though that ancient cross was worn and oxidized, ever-so-slightly tilting and partially uprooted, yet it stood there still. And I knew it had stood for so, so long—season after season after season after season. And that, I believe, is the lesson the Lord meant to teach me in that dream. This same cross, standing before me in the dead of winter, would also be there in the height of spring, the heat of summer, and the cool of autumn.

Thanks to that grace I have come to know, beloved, that this is our sure hope: The seasons change, but the God revealed in the face of the crucified Christ does not. And nothing, not even death, can separate us from Him.

Notes

Chapter 1 How Did I Get Here?

1. Russ Harris, *The Happiness Trap: How to Stop Struggling and Start Living* (Boston: Trumpeter Books, 2008), 41.

2. John Newton, "Amazing Grace," written 1779.

3. You can find hundreds of Dr. Price's sermons in the *Golden Grain* magazine, which began publication in the 1920s. Dr. Price passed away in 1947, but *Golden Grain* impacted many, long after his passing.

Chapter 2 Acceptance Is Not a Dirty Word

1. "My Way," Claude Francois, Gilles Thibaut, Jacques Revaux, Paul Anka, Warner Chappell Music France, Jeune Musique Editions, BMG Rights Management. Paul Anka rewrote an existing song; Frank Sinatra recorded and released it on the Reprise label in 1969.

2. C. G. Jung, *Modern Man in Search of a Soul* (San Diego, CA: Harvest, 1933), 234.

3. *APA Dictionary of Psychology*, s.v. "cognitive distortion," accessed December 8, 2021, https://dictionary.apa.org/cognitive-distortion.

4. Ibid.

5. For a list of cognitive distortions, see Christina Villarreal, "Fifteen Common Cognitive Distortions—How Our Thoughts Influence Our Mental Health," *Deep Mindset Coaching LLC*, March 30, 2010, https://drchristina villarreal.com/2010/03/30/15-common-cognitive-distortions-how-thoughts -influence-mental-health/.

6. *Merriam-Webster*, s.v. "what-if," Merriam-Webster.com, accessed December 8, 2021, https://www.merriam-webster.com/dictionary/what-ifs.

7. Matthew Tull, "What Is Trauma?" Verywell Mind, September 26, 2020, https://www.verywellmind.com/common-symptoms-after-a-traumatic-event-2797496.

8. Tull, "What Is Trauma?"

9. Tull, "What Is Trauma?"

Chapter 3 The Grunt Work of Getting Whole

1. The unconscious mind is "the region of the psyche containing memories, emotional conflicts, wishes, and repressed impulses that are not directly accessible to awareness but that have dynamic effects on thought and behavior." *APA Dictionary of Psychology*, s.v. "unconscious," accessed December 27, 2021, https://dictionary.apa.org/unconscious.

2. Karl Albrecht, "The (Only) Five Fears We All Share," *Psychology Today*, March 22, 2012, https://www.psychologytoday.com/ca/blog/brainsnacks/201203/the-only-5-fears-we-all-share.

3. David G. Benner, *Care of Souls: Revisioning Christian Nurture and Counsel* (Grand Rapids, MI: Baker Books, 1998), 65.

Chapter 4 Nothing's Perfect

1. Tasha Eurich, "What Self-Awareness Really Is (and How to Cultivate It)," *Harvard Business Review,* January 4, 2018, https://hbr.org/2018/01/what-self-awareness-really-is-and-how-to-cultivate-it.

2. Micah Abraham, "What Is Free Floating Anxiety?," *Calm Clinic*, October 10, 2020, https://www.calmclinic.com/anxiety/types/free-floating.

3. Saint Augustine, "Lord Jesus—Let Me Know Myself," accessed December 8, 2021, https://www.archspm.org/faith-and-discipleship/prayer/catholic-prayers/st-augustine-lord-jesus-let-me-know-myself.

Chapter 5 Perplexity, Apprehension, Anxiety

1. Dante, *Inferno* I.1, accessed December 9, 2021, https://www.poetryintranslation.com/PITBR/Italian/DantInf1to7.php#anchor_Toc64090910.

Chapter 6 Soul and Body

1. *Merriam-Webster*, s.v. "download," Merriam-Webster.com, accessed December 10, 2021, https://www.merriam-webster.com/dictionary/downloading.

Chapter 7 The Knot in My Stomach

1. *APA Dictionary of Psychology*, s.v. "cognitive distortion," accessed December 10, 2021, https://dictionary.apa.org/cognitive-distortion.

2. *APA Dictionary of Psychology*, s.v. "overgeneralization," accessed December 10, 2021, https://dictionary.apa.org/overgeneralization.

3. Tramain Hawkins, vocalist, "How I Got Over," lyrics by Clara Day, released 1986, track B1 on *The Search Is Over*, A&M Records, LP.

Chapter 9 A Dark Night of The Spirit

1. George Eldon Ladd, *A Theology of the New Testament* (Grand Rapids, MI: Eerdmans, 1974), 457.

2. Interestingly, this verse in Hebrews 4 is closely linked with a verse from one of the apocryphal books, 1 Enoch 9:5: "You have made everything and with you is the authority for everything. Everything is naked and open before your sight, and you see everything; and there is nothing which can hide itself from you," https://www.yahwehswordarchives.org/book-of-enoch/hanoch_enoch_08_09.htm.

Chapter 10 I Won't Complain. Or Will I?

1. Literally הַשָּׂטָן (*haśśāṭān*). See Stephen M. Hooks, *Job* (Joplin, MO: College Press Pub., 2006), 61. While most translations leave out the definite article, in the Hebrew it is indeed there. In other words, at this stage in biblical history, the adversary isn't named specifically Satan. Rather, the definite article implies that this angelic creature serves as a prosecuting attorney with sinister motives.

2. The book of Job was probably written about a thousand years before Jesus came on the scene. Just to give you a sense of time and history, this is about the same time that Samuel was prophet in Israel, and Saul and David were alive. By the time the story was told, the sons of Esau had spread out in the eastern direction. And some argue that Job was written by a descendant of Esau, perhaps by an Egyptian or Mesopotamian. Think about what it would mean if the book of Job was not written by an Israelite (or even about an Israelite) yet showed up in the Hebrew canon.

3. Not all of Israel broke the covenant. Yet God dealt with them as one people, so that when judgment came, even the righteous had to endure Yahweh's chastenings. Those chastenings served a different purpose for the remnant than for the rebellious. The remnant learned from the sufferings, even though they wrestled with justice issues and wondered why they had to endure what they endured. The rebels learned nothing. They had already been worshiping the gods of Babylon, the Baals, long before Nebuchadnezzar ransacked Jerusalem, destroyed its walls, burned it to the ground, destroyed the Temple, took all the holy furnishings into Babylon, and placed them in their temple (bringing God's holy utensils into a defiled atmosphere).

4. Paul Jones recorded this early in 1982, but it seems to have been originally written by Don Johnson in 1977 and recorded with a country-and-western feel. Originally, it was titled "I Can't Complain." See https://youtu.be/cLhq715nfqg.

5. To watch a recording of one of Bishop Abney's performances, go to https://youtu.be/NZCOpmd9ILM.

6. Don H. Johnson, "I Won't Complain," Gospel Lyrics, accessed December 27, 2021, https://gospellyrics.info/2007/08/17/i-won-t-complain/.

Chapter 11 Power and Powerlessness

1. As examples, see Genesis 18:25; Exodus 20:5–6; 32:33–34; Leviticus 26:23–25; Deuteronomy 7:9–10; 32:3–4, 35, 41–43; 2 Chronicles 12:1–6; Psalm 58:10–11; Proverbs 24:12; Isaiah 1:24; Jeremiah 5:7–9.

Chapter 12 Fear and Hope

1. Francis I. Andersen, *Job: An Introduction and Commentary* (Downers Grove, IL: InterVarsity, 1997), 117.

2. John E. Hartley, *The Book of Job* (Grand Rapids, MI: Eerdmans, 1988), 100.

3. Lit. ἐνθύμησις, εως f; νόημαᵇ, τος n; διάνοιαᶜ, ας f; διανόημα, τος n: the content of thinking and reasoning—"thought, what is thought, opinion." ἐνθύμησις: ἰδὼν ὁ Ἰησοῦς τὰς ἐνθυμήσεις αὐτῶν "Jesus knew what they were thinking," Matthew 9:4; χαράγματι τέχνης καὶ ἐνθυμήσεως ἀνθρώπου "formed by the skill and thought of people," Acts 17:29. Louw and Nida, *Greek-English Lexicon of the New Testament: Based on Semantic Domains* (New York: United Bible Societies, 1996), 350–51.

4. Lit. μεθοδεία, ας f: crafty scheming with the intent to deceive—"deceit, scheming." πρὸς τὸ δύνασθαι ὑμᾶς στῆναι πρὸς τὰς μεθοδείας τοῦ διαβόλου "so that you can stand up against the Devil's scheming." Louw and Nida, *Greek-English Lexicon of the New Testament*, 759.

5. T. Austin-Sparks, "Ascension and Glory," *Incorporated into Christ*, accessed December 15, 2021, https://www.austin-sparks.net/english/books /004849.html.

6. Austin-Sparks, "Ascension and Glory."

7. The prologue of Job, as we have seen, refers to the heavenly council. Jeremiah refers to it as well (see Jeremiah 23:18).

8. That word for trial implies "to tempt, to trap, to lead into temptation." πειράζως; ἐκπειράζως; πειρασμόςb, οῦ m: to endeavor or attempt to cause someone to sin—"to tempt, to trap, to lead into temptation, temptation." πειράζως: ἦν ἐν τῇ ἐρήμῳ τεσσεράκοντα ἡμέρας πειραζόμενος ὑπὸ τοῦ Σατανᾶ "he stayed for forty days in the desert and Satan tried to make him sin," Mark 1:13. In translating expressions involving tempting or trying, it is necessary in a number of languages to indicate clearly whether or not the temptations succeeded. It may not be sufficient in Mark 1:13, therefore, to simply say, "Satan tempted him"; in fact, in some instances it may be necessary to make the failure of the temptation quite specific, for example, "Satan tried to make Jesus sin, but was not successful." Louw and Nida, *Greek-English Lexicon of the New Testament*, 774.

9. On this point, I agree with John Wesley's view of divine sovereignty and reject completely John Calvin's and Theodore Beza's teachings on predestination, as well as their idea of "double predestination."

10. In future studies, there is a discipline known as "horizon scanning." This involves gathering all the information one has related to trends and trajectories of what is emerging in various domains in current reality in order to anticipate, as well as possible, the future prior to its arrival. It isn't about treating the future with crystal-ball thinking. It is rooted in raw data and the arc of historical trends and patterns that repeat themselves predictably over the course of time, both long-term and short-term. Within future studies, there are four primary ways to categorize the future: the *plausible* future, the *probable* future, the *possible* future, and the *preferred* future. Remember the old saying, "Expect the unexpected"? It brings us to another dynamic of the future identified by future studies, commonly called the "wild card" event. Nassim Nicholas Taleb in his best-selling book renamed it the "black swan" event. This is an event you cannot see coming, though you do have to learn to make room for it to happen because its impact is enormous. The wild card is always unlikely, but when it occurs it literally changes the rules of the game. After such events our minds are thrown into rationalization mode. In order to regain some sense of control, we try desperately to convince ourselves that we could have seen it coming and didn't because we weren't paying attention. As I've said many times in this book, I did not see the bus coming, and if I had, I'd have gotten out of the way. The truth is, however, I could not have seen it coming. I had to learn not to blame myself for something that was truly beyond my control.

11. Hooks, *Job*, 72–73.

Epilogue Daring to Dream

1. One of the oldest surviving stone crosses is in Donegal, Ireland, and is known as St. Patrick's Cross. According to Irish tradition, St. Patrick founded a monastery there in the fifth century.

Dr. Mark Chironna is a lifelong learner who studies for the sake of his call: to serve Christ by bringing his saving, healing, and empowering truth to everyday people. All people are created in the image of God, yet everyone faces adversity, disappointment, and difficulty. Knowing this, Dr. Chironna preaches, teaches, speaks, and writes about the gospel and shares transparently about his own difficult seasons. He believes that to know and love Christ is to honor and understand not only the divine destiny of every human being but also the sufferings that are part of the human condition. Because of this, he labors to equip others. His hope is that Christ might be fully formed in them, for their benefit and God's glory.

Dr. Chironna holds a holistic view of spirituality, psychology, and theology. He does not see people as segmented beings but as integrated persons for whom the spiritual, physical, emotional, and psychological are inseparable. His view is not primarily philosophical but theological. He therefore emphasizes orthodoxy, sound teaching, and adherence to the Great Tradition that has guided the Church through the millennia. Dr. Chironna's extensive multidisciplinary training and experience includes board-certified coaching, a master's degree in psychology, a doctoral degree in applied semiotics and future leadership studies, and a soon-to-be-completed PhD in theology at the University of Birmingham (UK). For Dr. Chironna, these endeavors are more than theoretical and academic; they are a practical part of his mission to serve others, and particularly the Body of Christ.

In addition to pastoring the flock at Church on the Living Edge in Orlando, Florida, Dr. Chironna is the presiding bishop of Legacy Edge Alliance, a worldwide fellowship of senior apostolic leaders and churches. He is also the bishop protector of the Order of St. Maximus the Confessor, an order recently inaugurated by the International Communion of Charismatic Churches and devoted to the furthering of sound prophetic practice. His outreach includes a weekly television program, *On the Living Edge*, as well as *The Edge Podcast* and Facebook, Twitter, and Instagram platforms. Dr. Chironna and his wife, Pastor Ruth Chironna, have two grown sons and four grandchildren.

On the Living Edge, Daystar Television, Thursdays,
    10:30 p.m.
The Edge Podcast, available on all platforms
dr.markchironna
@markchironna
www.markchironna.com